KETO DIET | LOW CARB | MEDITERRANEAN DIET | INTERMITTENT FASTING

The 4 in 1 Weight Loss Cookbook with Healthy and Delicious Recipes for Every Day incl. Meal Planner and 30 Days Diet Plan

Adam K. Parker

Copyright © [2019] [Adam K. Parker]]

All rights reserved

All rights for this book here presented belong exclusively to the author.
Usage or reproduction of the text is forbidden and requires a clear consent of the author in case of expectations.

ISBN: 9798671066685

TABLE OF CONTENTS

Exclusive Bonus! 11
Introduction 13
    Health Benefits of Weight Loss 14
        Why Obesity is a Health Hazard 15
    Unsuitable Methods to Lose Weight 16
KETO DIET 19
What Exactly Is the Keto Diet? 21
What are the Benefits of the Keto Diet 23
    Losing weight healthily 23
    Lowers Blood Sugar 23
    Focus and Brain Health 23
    Feel Fuller for Longer 24
    Epilepsy 24
    Blood Pressure and Cholesterol Reductions 24
    Acne 24
How to lose weight effectively with the Keto Diet 25
    Foods to avoid include: 25
    Foods you're allowed to eat, EAT AND EAT SOME MORE! 26
How to Prepare for the Keto Diet 29
    Reaching Ketosis 29
    Are you in Ketosis? 30
    The Keto Flu 30
RECIPES 33
    Breakfast 34
        Chicken and Waffle Sandwiches 35
        Breakfast Bowl 37
        Blueberry Pancake Bites 39
        Stuffed Peppers 40
        Spicy Eggs and Cheesy Hash 41

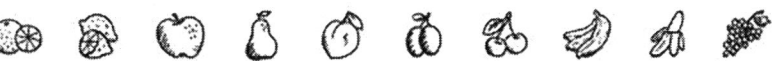

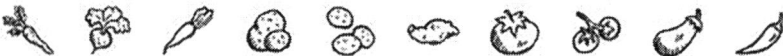

Faux-Tatoe Bubble and Squeak	43
Bacon Bagels	45
Ricotta and Blueberry Pancakes	47
Chorizo Baked Eggs	48
Eggs Benedict Casserole	49

Exclusive Bonus! 51

Lunch 52
- Tuna and Pesto Salad 53
- Steak and Mushroom Stroganoff 54
- Cheesy Beer Soup 55
- Salmon Burgers on Cedar Plank 57
- Bacon Cheeseburger Kebabs 59
- Taco-Stuffed Avos 61
- Bacon Salad with Kale 63
- Eggs Benedict Salad with Bacon 64
- Pressed Halloumi with Blackberry, Basil and Spinach 65

Dinner 66
- In-A-Skillet Philly Cheesesteak 67
- Instant Pot Faux-Lasagna 68
- Chicken Salad with Bacon 69
- Salisbury Steak and Cauli Mash 70
- Faux Crab Cakes 72
- Mushroom Steaks with Avo Salsa 73
- Creamy Spinach Alfredo with Zucchini Curls 74
- Chicken Meatloaf Cupcakes 76
- Shrimp and Caulirice 78

Desserts and Snacks 80
- Coconut Avocado Smoothie 81
- Neapolitan Chia Dessert 82
- Almond and Coconut Cookies 83
- Coconut Avo Ice Cream 84
- CocoChoc Mug Cake 85

14 Day Meal Plan 87

5 Quick Tips to Losing Weight with Keto 105

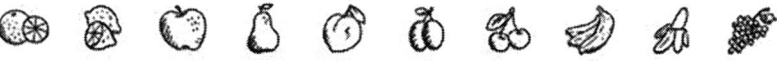

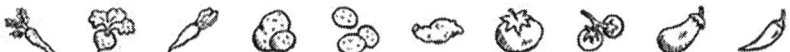

Exclusive Bonus!	106
Low Carb	107
Introduction	109
What is Low Carb?	109
History of Low Carb	110
Everything You Need to Know About Carbs	110
What Happens in Our Body?	113
Used for Fuel	113
Saved for Later	114
Stored as Fat	114
Is Low Carb Really Healthy?	115
Decrease Overall Appetite	115
More Weight Loss at First	115
More Fat is Lost from Abdomen Area	116
Drastic Reduction in Triglycerides	116
"Good" HDL Cholesterol Increases	117
"Bad" LDL Cholesterol Decreases	117
Reduction in Insulin and Blood Sugar Levels	117
Decrease Blood Pressure	118
Treats Several Brain Disorders	118
What Should I Avoid?	121
Breads/Grains	121
Some Fruits	122
Starchy Veggies	122
Pasta	123
Breakfast Cereal	123
Beer	124
Sweetened Yogurt	124
Juice	125
Low-Fat/Fat-Free Salad Dressings	125
Beans/Legumes	126
Honey/Sugar (any kind)	126
Chips/Crackers	127
Milk	127

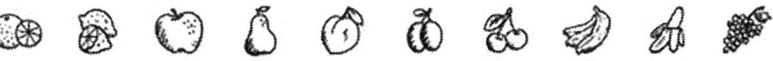

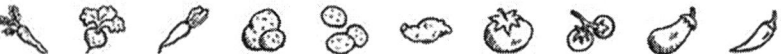

Gluten-Free Baked Goods	127
What am I Allowed to Eat?	129
Meat	129
Fish/Seafood	129
Eggs	129
Natural Fats/High-Fat Sauces	130
Veggies	130
Dairy	130
Nuts	130
Berries	131
Drinks	131
Celebrations/Special Events	131
How Many Carbs Should I Consume Each Day?	133
How to Get Started on a Low Carb Eating Plan	135
Reduce Carb Consumption	135
Stay Full & Satisfied	137
Choose a Diet You Can Stick With Long-Term	138
Atkins	138
South Beach Diet	139
Ketogenic Diet	140
Dukan Diet	140
Paleo Diet	140
Stay Healthy & Motivated	141
Low Carb Recipes	143
Low Carb Breakfast Recipes	144
Goat Cheese & Herb Omelet	145
Frittata with Spinach & Goat Cheese	146
Fried Egg Sandwich	147
Spinach Quiche (No Crust)	148
Egg & Cheese Boats	149
Sausage Casserole	150
Oven Scrambled Eggs	151
Oven-Baked Denver Omelet	152
Ham, Cheese, & Hashbrown Casserole	153

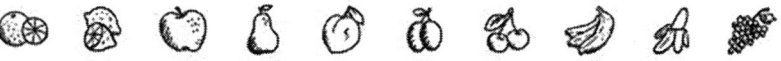

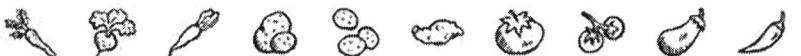

French Toast	154
Low Carb Lunch Recipes	155
Chipped Beef on Toast	156
Low Carb Burger	157
Beef Dip Sandwich	158
Garlic Salmon	159
Bacon & Feta Stuffed Chicken Breasts	160
Turkey Burgers with Feta Cheese	161
Ham & Cheese Rolls	162
BBQ Bacon Shrimp	163
Grilled Mushrooms	164
Grilled Tandoori Chicken	165
Meatballs w/ Sweet & Sour Sauce	167
Herby Lemon Chicken	168
Gyro Burger	169
Low Carb Dinner Recipes	170
Lasagna Stuffed Peppers	171
Chicken Cacciatore	172
Roast Chicken w/ Lemon & Carrots	173
Stuffed Summer Squash	175
Candied Bacon Chicken with Cauliflower Rice & Pecans	176
Lettuce Wraps	178
Beef Slaw	179
Lasagna Stuffed Mushrooms	180
Sweet Potato Carbonara with Mushrooms & Spinach	181
Grilled Salmon Wraps	183
Parmesan Tilapia	184
Pork Chops with Mushroom Sauce	185
Low Carb Dessert Recipes	186
Almond-Raspberry Cupcakes	187
Chocolate-Peanut Butter Whip	189
Pumpkin Pecan Cheesecake	190
Vanilla Almond Butter Cookies	192
Tiramisu Cupcakes	193
Low Carb Snack Recipes	195
Blackberry-Coconut Fat Bombs	196

    Pizza Bites 197
    Salt & Vinegar Zucchini Chips 199
    Chocolate Quinoa Bites..200
    Pepper Nachos 201
  Low Carb Smoothie Recipes 202
    Chocolate-Avocado Smoothie...203
    Very Berry Smoothie 204
    Chocolate Peanut Butter Smoothie 205
    Coffee Smoothie 206
    Avocado/Spinach/Strawberry Smoothie 207

Bonus: 10 Ways to Lose Weight Fast 209
  Begin Your Day with Warm Lemon Water.....................................209
  Get at least 30 mins of Physical Activity Daily................................209
  Be Sure to Get Your Fiber 210
  Consume Healthy Protein Sources at Every Meal 210
  Pay Attention to What You're Eating..210
  Choose Healthy Snacks...210
  Discover Healthy Alternatives to Your Favorite Treats 210
  Learn to Manage Your Stress...211
  Kick Those Bad Habits..211
  Make a Plan to be Successful 211

Intermittent Fasting..213

Intermittent Fasting and How it Works 215
    The 16:8 Method 220
    The 5:2 Method 221

Mediterranean Diet..223

Mediterranean Diet Cookbook..225
  What is the Mediterranean Diet? 225
  How to Get Started 226

Recipes...227
  Breakfast..228
    Avocado Toast Caprese Style..229
    Frittata w/ Asparagus, Mushroom, & Goat Cheese.....................230
    Poached Egg with Greens & White Beans 232

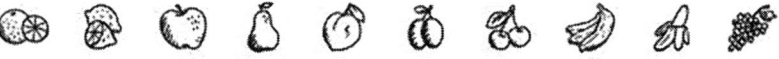

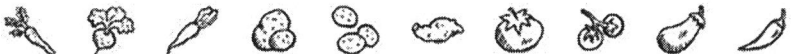

    Start Your Morning Right Grain Salad 234
    Easy Muesli 236
Meat 237
    Grilled Balsamic Chicken w/ Olive Tapenade 238
    Pork Scaloppini w/ Lemon and Capers 240
    Greek Turkey Burgers 242
    Pomegranate Citrus Glazed Duck Breast 244
    Skewered Beef w/ Garlic White Bean Sauce 246
    Chicken Kebabs 248
    Chicken w/ Tomato and Balsamic Sauce 250
    Mediterranean Spaghetti Squash w/ Turkey 252
    Boneless Pork Chops w/ Vegetables 254
    Garlic Steak w/ Warm Spinach 256
Fish & Seafood 257
    Shrimp Piccata w/ Zucchini Noodles 258
    Walnut Crusted Salmon 259
    Greek Baked Shrimp 260
    Bass w/ Tomatoes and Olives 261
    Couscous w/ Tuna 262
    Parmesan Pesto Tilapia 263
    Honey Mustard Salmon 264
Vegetables 265
    Stuffed Portobello Mushrooms Caprese Style 266
    Zucchini Lasagna Rolls 267
    Stuffed Sweet Potatoes 268
    Roasted Stuffed Eggplant 269
    Slow Cooker Minestrone 271
Salad 273
    Avocado Caprese Salad 274
    Chickpea and Herb Salad 275
    Sun-Dried Tomato and Feta Couscous Salad 276
    Greek Salad w/ Avocado 277
    Arugula Salad w/ Parmesan 278
Snacks & Desserts 279
    No-Bake Mint Chip Cookies 280
    Grain-Free Hummingbird Cake 281

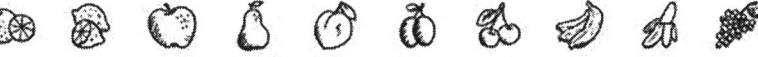

    Pumpkin Chia Seed Pudding..282
    Baked Zucchini Chips..283
    Sun-Dried Tomato and Goat Cheese Spread......................................284

30 Days Lose Weight Challenge..285

Disclaimer..320

EXCLUSIVE BONUS!

Get Keto Audiobook for FREE NOW!*

*The Ultimate Keto Diet Guide 2019-2020:
How to Loose weight with Quick and Easy Steps*

SCAN ME

or go to

www.free-keto.co.uk

*Listen free for 30 Days on Audible (for new members only)

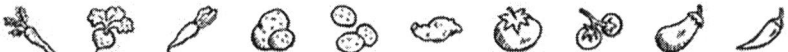

Introduction

Diet. It has become a nasty word in the minds of many, and this is unfortunate. In ancient Greek, where the word **diet** originates, it meant *a mode of living*. Diet simply means the kinds of food that a person, animal, or community habitually eats. It also carries the definition of a special course of food to which a person restricts themselves, either for medical reasons or to lose weight. As a verb, diet appears in the dictionary as "restrict oneself to small amounts or special kinds of food in order to lose weight."

In a negative sense, the word *diet* has come to suggest a regime for the purpose of weight loss. Should we not aspire to return to the original derivation as the ancients intended? It seems preferential to approach our diets as a more holistic way of life and health. A mode of living is surely more appealing than an imposed regime.

Not every person is the same, and indeed age, health concerns, culture and genetics do all contribute to weight and body structure. They also play significant roles in the body's dynamics and development. It must be accepted that not all people can have similar bodies by following the same diet. Menopausal women must adapt their diet according to a decreased metabolic rate and metabolism. Triathletes will need a higher protein intake. Pregnant and breastfeeding women must ensure suitable nourishment to adapt to also nourishing the baby. Cultures differ in regional diets: divergences include vegetarians, teetotallers, enthusiastic meat-eaters, and many others.

A flexible eating plan is more embracing than restrictive in the sense that it does not forbid certain foods or food groups. A flexible diet rather embraces variety: foods from each major food group, incorporating fruits, vegetables, dairy products, whole grains, nuts, seeds, and lean protein sources. Liberating rather than constricting is a better way to live.

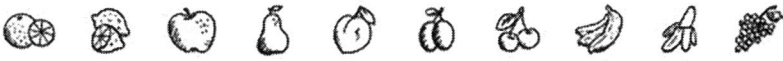

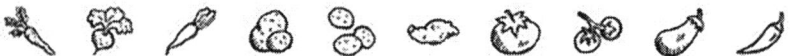

Health Benefits of Weight Loss

Obesity is only one of the dangers behind carrying that extra weight, especially when the extra weight is in certain parts of your body. It stands to reason that not carrying one's ideal personal weight will lead to a certain level of discomfort, but it can also be detrimental to health and wellbeing.

Obesity refers to excess body fat. BMI or Body Mass Index does not measure body fat directly but uses standard weight status categories to track weight standing. It does not account for age, sex, ethnicity, or muscle mass in adults. A certain amount of body fat is necessary for heat insulation, energy storage, and similar functions, and BMI therefore ranges as follows:

Normal weight: BMI of 18.5 to 24.9

Overweight: BMI of 25 to 29.9

Obese: BMI over 30

Morbidly obese: BMI over 40

Adiposity is a condition of being obese or severely overweight. The body adiposity index (BAI) differs from BMI in that it does not consider weight but is measured using height and hip circumference.

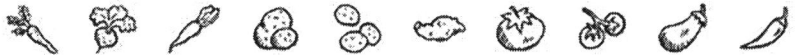

WHY OBESITY IS A HEALTH HAZARD

Obesity is a chronic medical disease that can lead to chronic illnesses, increased risk of many serious diseases and adverse health conditions, including:

Type 2 diabetes
Coronary heart disease
Body pain and difficulty with physical functioning
Osteoarthritis
Sleep apnoea
Mortality
Stroke
High blood pressure (Hypertension)
Gallbladder disease
High LDL cholesterol
Low HDL cholesterol
Breathing problems
Cancers such as breast, colon, liver, endometrial, kidney, and gallbladder
Clinical depression
Anxiety
Certain mental disorders

Obesity has a significant relapse rate and is hard to treat, with many regaining any weight loss achieved within five years. Although crash diets and medication can help, a short-term "fix" is not the answer. Obesity should ideally be treated through a lifelong commitment to regular exercise and/or increased physical activity, and correct eating habits.

Of course all aspects of the dangers of weight cannot be satisfactorily dealt with here, but all efforts will be made to at least touch on those which are most prevalent.

The sugar-belly is frequently a bug-bear for most people battling weight or poor body image. We all know what visceral fat looks like, but the manner in which the muffin

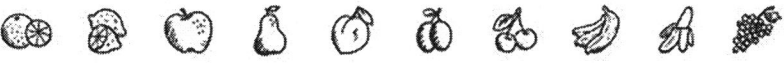

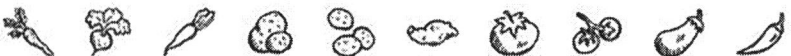

top develops is very interesting to understand. It all starts with the body balancing glucose and insulin. Glucose is the body and brain's energy source. Insulin is released by the pancreas to transport the glucose from the blood stream to the muscle and brain cells. The more glucose you pump into your body, the more insulin it needs to process it, and this is the beginning of what will become belly fat.

Food is digested into glucose from carbohydrates; amino acids from protein and fatty acids from fat. Carbohydrates however are not all digested in the same way. Some break down quickly, others take a while longer, and fibrous carbohydrates don't break down at all. Sugar is one that is digested the quickest, along with refined carbohydrates – which for ease of reference is all the white processed foods such as white flour, pasta and white bread. These cause a spike in blood-glucose that needs a rush of insulin to process. All that insulin hanging about is much like a tattoo in that it's way easier to get than to get rid of. It leads to the body storing more fat than it typically would and also prevents it using fat for energy between meals. It becomes a vicious circle of feeling hungry because your stored fat is not being used as fuel, over-producing insulin, and storing yet more fat.

The real villain in this fat tale is fructose. The human body was designed to process fructose in small amounts because back when we roamed the earth hunting and gathering, it took a while to find berries and fruit and honey in the wild. Nowadays sugar is freely available in its most malevolent form, and it swells our tummies and ruins our health.

Fat mass loss will benefit improving risk factors linked to obesity no matter the region of the body from which it is lost. Total fat mass loss is best for overall health. Losing fat mass reduces symptoms of chronic diseases as well as the danger of getting associated diseases.

Unsuitable Methods to Lose Weight

While a healthy weight becomes crucial for longevity, certain tried and tested means to lose weight throughout human history have proven less than ideal. Some of these may

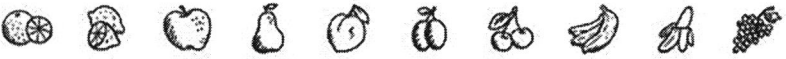

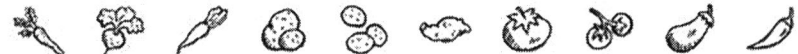

seem ridiculous, but the fact remains that there is always someone out there willing to push the boundaries of normal to reach their goals. These are but a few:

The vinegar diet promoted consuming lashings of vinegar, together with a raw egg and a cuppa tea, which would cause purging, loss of appetite and consequently, weight. The legacy persists past its heyday in the 1820 in current claims that apple cider vinegar can help with weight loss. Copious consumption of vinegar could potentially irritate the stomach lining, cause a potassium imbalance, and erode tooth enamel, which does not warrant the possible weight benefits.

The cabbage soup diet is definitely not a long-term option, although it quite possibly will shed flab and do away with bloating for a fast result. The diet is incredibly restrictive, limited to a week of cabbage soup and limited meals only. It lacks vital nutrients, including carbohydrates and healthy fats and is very much the epitome of a yo-yo fad diet which will only cause chaos metabolically. Initial weight loss will surely be followed by exponentially more weight gain once normal eating is resumed.

The grapefruit juice diet is dangerous in that it severely restricts calorie intake. While adding the obligatory half grapefruit or glass of freshly squeezed grapefruit juice to every meal has no harmful effects per se, limiting calories to 1000 per day makes this a fad. It should also be noted that grapefruit may clash with certain medications.

Starvation diets have long term and far reaching negative effects in the body. Body composition describes the components of a human body, which are both fat and fat-free mass. Fat-free mass comprises all that is NOT fat. These are water, protein (lean muscle, organs), minerals (bones and iron in the blood). Lean body mass, a component of body composition, is ascertained through the deducting body fat figure from total body weight. Changing body composition must be done through maintaining lean body mass while reducing fat mass, and not just concentrating on weight loss. Starvation causes significant loss of lean body mass and lean muscle mass (water, organs, bones). Results include decreased bone density, changes in metabolism, reduced lean muscle, decreased strength, and susceptibility to injury. Weight loss is usually followed by

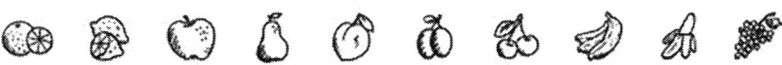

significant weight gain within 8 years, as well as increasing the probability of the onset of such eating disorders as bulimia or anorexia.

KETO DIET

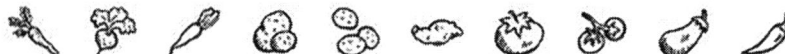

What Exactly Is the Keto Diet?

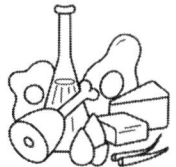

By now everyone has heard the term "keto diet", but what exactly is it and does it really work? Keto, short for ketogenic, is basically a low-carb, high-fat diet, where you eat foods that have a high good fat content and low carbohydrate content. You may have heard of similar diets, like banting for example. Your body's fuel source usually comes from glucose, also known as blood sugar, but we all know that if our blood sugar levels get too high, we run the risk of developing Type 2 Diabetes. Keto actually allows your body to create an alternative fuel source, called ketones. Carbohydrates convert into glucose for energy, but when you reduce your carb intake; your liver begins converting fats into ketones, providing you, especially your brain, with essential energy. When you are following the keto diet, your body changes from running on carbs, to running on fats. Your body is now in a state known as ketosis, and is constantly burning fats for energy. Not only is this great news a bonus for weight watchers, but studies have shown that this food lifestyle can even reverse Type 2 diabetes! Other benefits include staying full for longer, so you stop reaching for that sneaky chocolate for a quick snack. Due to these benefits, many doctors are encouraging patients to try their hand at following the keto diet.

There are a few different styles of the keto diet, aimed at different types of people. The Cycilcal and Targeted Keto Diets are mostly utilized by athletes and bodybuilders, as they are not based on a lifestyle change, but shorter periods of quick dieting. The most common forms of the keto diets are the Standard and the High-Protein Keto Diets. These are the ones that are encouraged by doctors, especially for patients that need to consider their blood sugar levels. The Standard and High-protein keto diets have

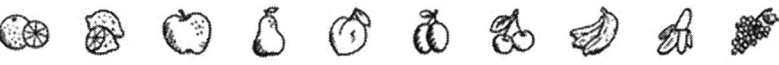

minute differences, in that the High-protein diet simply incorporates less fat and more protein than the Standard version. The choice of which one suits you best, is entirely up to you. Typically the Standard one uses 75% of fats, 20% of protein and 5% of carbs, whereas the High-protein one uses 60% of fats, 35% of protein and 5% of carbs.

What are the Benefits of the Keto Diet

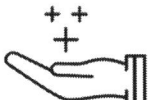

Losing weight healthily

As we have mentioned, one major benefit to this diet is weight loss and doing it all in a healthy manner. Because your fat-storing hormone (insulin) levels drop, your body becomes a fat-burning machine! Yes, you still have to work at it and dedicate yourself to eating correctly, but what could be better than being slimmer and healthier all at once?!

Lowers Blood Sugar

Due to the types of food you will eat, the keto diet naturally reduces the blood sugar levels. Some studies have found that the keto diet is the most effective way to control, prevent and even reverse Type 2 diabetes. If you have been diagnosed with Type 2 diabetes, or are even pre-diabetic, you really should consider giving the keto diet a chance.

Focus and Brain Health

Many people in high pressure jobs use the keto diet to improve their brain health and its ability to keep you focussed and energized. Ketones are a fantastic brain fuel source. Lowering your carbs, helps limit you from having blood sugar spikes. Combining the two improves concentration and keeps you alert.

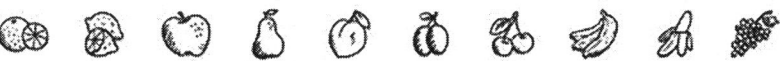

Feel Fuller for Longer

The foods you eat on the keto diet are more satisfying due to the high fat content, and they help you feel full for longer periods. Say you have breakfast around 7am, instead of feeling peckish again at 10am, you can actually continue through until lunch time.

Epilepsy

Keto was actually introduced in the early 1900's, as a successful treatment for epilepsy in children and is still being prescribed today. Epilepsy sufferers who employ the keto diet, report using fewer medicines as a result.

Blood Pressure and Cholesterol Reductions

Many studies have shown significant improvements in followers of the keto diet, to their triglyceride and cholesterol levels, and their blood pressure. These ailments often are associated with heart problems. Blood pressure is also affected by weight, so the weight loss that comes naturally with keto, is an added bonus to high blood pressure sufferers.

Acne

Indeed not one you would usually consider, but skin has always seen noticeable improvements when following a low-carb high-fat diet. If you're showing signs of acne or general skin issues, perhaps consider your diet, especially if you're currently eating way too many fast and sugary foods.

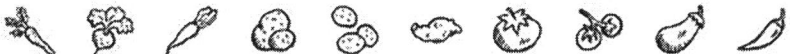

How to lose weight effectively with the Keto Diet

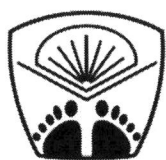

Sick of having to watch what you eat, counting calories and weighing your food, and yet still starving an hour later? Some studies have shown that people following the oft recommended low-fat diet, tend to lose weight, but put it all back on again. Similar studies following keto dieters have found that those dieters have lost considerably more weight. Also they are not starving themselves and have a general improved outlook, both outside with weight loss and inside with improved cholesterol and / or blood sugar. So what's the secret? And how can the keto diet benefit you? Firstly, you need to know which foods you cannot have and eliminate them completely from your diet. It helps to get rid of them from your kitchen entirely, so you're not even tempted. Now, don't be upset when you read this list. Yes, you're going to be giving up a LOT! But, just think about ALL those gains like weight loss (new wardrobe!), healthy brain and heart, more energy, and potentially no more Type 2 diabetes if you're a sufferer.

Foods to avoid include:

- ✓ Sugary foods: This is an obvious one of course, and covers things like soda, fruit juice (even the 100% ones!), cake, ice cream, sweets and candy. Smoothies too, if you haven't made them yourself.

- ✓ Starches and grains: Anything made with wheat including pasta, rice, breakfast cereals, bread, etc. An easy way to look at something with grains is to ask if it was made with white flour. If yes, then it's off your list.

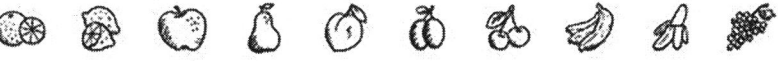

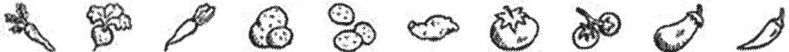

- ✓ Fruit: Shocker, yes, but not all fruit is off limits. Berries like strawberries, blueberries and even avocados (YES!) are allowed in proportion. Other fruit is off limits because of the carbs in them and they have surprisingly loads.

- ✓ Beans and legumes: Peas, beans, chickpeas, etc. Note that peanuts are included in this section, as they are actually legumes and not nuts.

- ✓ Root vegetables: Too many carbs in potatoes, carrots, yams and the like.

- ✓ Diet / low-fat / sugar-free products: Don't be fooled! These products are highly processed and often high in sugar alternatives and carbs. These can have an adverse affect on your ketone levels and make it harder for you to reach ketosis.

- ✓ Sauces and condiments: Mostly contain lots of sugar and bad fats.

- ✓ Bad fats: These are things like cooking oil (sunflower, canola, vegetable), margarine and mayonnaise.

- ✓ Alcohol: Again, too many carbs. If you want to lose that beer belly, you have to get rid of the beer!

Foods you're allowed to eat, EAT AND EAT SOME MORE!

- ✓ Meat: All meat! Beef, chicken, pork, fish, lamb, rabbit, and more! YES! Bring on that steak!

- ✓ Leafy Greens and above-ground vegetables: kale, lettuce, cauliflower. If you do not have to dig it up to eat it, you can eat it!

- ✓ Dairy with high-fat content: whole milk, hard cheese, fresh cream, eggs. Skip that 2% and go for the full cream milk!

- ✓ Seeds and nuts: cashews, macadamias, sunflower seeds, chia seeds. Excellent snackage material here!

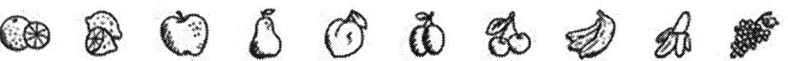

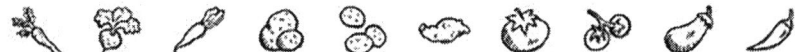

- Berries: Strawberries, raspberries, blueberries, and the best berry of all: the Avocado!

- Sweeteners: Sugar alternatives include erythritol, stevia (which is found in some soft drinks now), xylitol and monk fruit. Be warned though, that if you have pets in the house, you are strongly discouraged from using xylitol, as it is lethal for them.

- Other good fats: Olive oil (preferably extra-virgin), coconut oil, high-fat salad dressings, butter, nut butter.

- Condiments: Not all condiments are banned. Salt, pepper, spiced and herbs are allowed.

See, it's not all bad, right? And we all know that when you have to diet, whether to lose a few pounds or just to get healthier, sacrifices have to be made. With keto, all you need to remember is the food must be high in fats, middle-ground in proteins, and low in carbohydrates. If you're planning on using the Standard keto version, make your per day nutrient intake around 70% high-fat, 25% protein and the remaining 5% carbs. Lowering your carbohydrate intake will improve overall results. Proteins should always been eaten as needed, and the fats filling in all the gaps for the remainder of your day. With weight loss, it's a good trick to note your total carbohydrates and your net carbohydrates. To calculate your net carbs, simply take the total carbs of an item and subtract the total fiber. It is recommended that total carbs per day are kept below 35g and net carbs, ideally, below 20g per day.

In the beginning of getting used to this new lifestyle, you may find yourself getting hungry during the day. Snacking on nuts, seeds, or even some peanut butter should help keep the temptations away. Bear in mind that snacking can slow down your weight loss. If you're weighing yourself periodically and notice very little has changed, go through your day and see how much snacking you have done and decide to either increase the size of a meal, or stop snacking cold turkey.

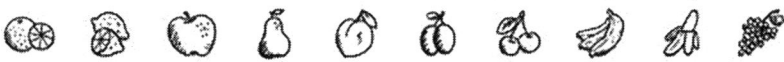

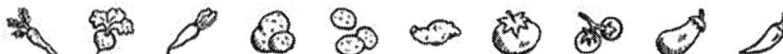

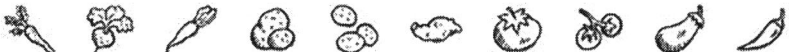

How to Prepare for the Keto Diet

Reaching Ketosis

To get the maximum out of the keto diet and all that fat burning going, you need to reach the ketosis stage. Achieving this is quite straightforward, but can seem complicated, so here's a simplified list to get you going:

1. **Limit your carb intake**: Limit all carbs, both total and net carbs. Keeping them below the 35g (total carbs) and 25g (net carbs) recommended limits, will help you to get to the ketosis stage faster.
2. **Limit your protein intake**: Eating too much protein can cause lower levels of ketosis. For weight loss, you ideally need to eat between 0.6g – 0.8g of proteins per pound lean body mass.
3. **Don't stress about fat!** Eating fats is the main source of energy on the keto diet, so ensure you're getting enough. Do not starve yourself!
4. **Drink plenty of water!** Staying hydrated is vital to your body and helps control any hunger pangs too. Try to drink about 2 liters / 0.5 gallons of water per day.
5. **Snacking:** Limit the snacking as it can slow down the process. It also reduces the number of insulin spikes, which elevates your blood sugar levels.
6. **Consider fasting:** A good tool to increase ketone levels is to fast intermittently. This in no way means starving yourself, in the traditional sense of fasting, but simply cutting out a meal here or there. Note thought that fasting is not for everyone, so if you can't, don't.

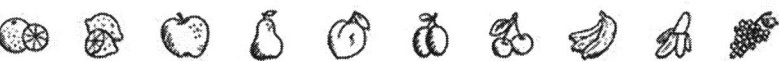

7. **Exercise:** ah the dreaded exercise. We know that getting exercise is good for us, but not all of us are cut out for going to the gym. If you prefer a more sedentary exercise regime, add in a short walk to help the ketosis along.
8. **Become a label reader:** Some products are designed to catch your eye, as being beneficial to the dieter. This is NOT always the case. Be sure to read the labels carefully and you will be surprised at how many hidden carbs are in so-called diet-friendly products.

Are you in Ketosis?

There are various products on offer, that can tell you if you're in the ketosis stage, but most of them are expensive and just inaccurate. The following list of things should give you a good indication of whether you are in ketosis:

1. **Needing to urinate more:** The keto diet naturally makes you want to use the bathroom more often.
2. **Dry Mouth:** The more you wee, the more you will get thirsty. Ensure you're drinking plenty of water.
3. **Bad breath:** Not a pleasant thought or what anyone would want to experience. The good thing is that this does not last forever. Just keep some sugar-free (check the labels!) gum nearby, in case you're concerned.
4. **Limited hunger and Energy Boosts:** Once you get into ketosis, you may notice that you can survive longer between meals and have more energy.

The Keto Flu

While the keto diet is safe for the majority of people, there are some undesirable side effects. We've already mentioned the bad breath, but the one you need to be on the lookout for is the keto flu, also known as carb flu. The symptoms of keto flu can feel similar to actual flu, but are caused by the body trying to adapt to the new eating lifestyle. The drastic reduction of carbohydrate intake shocks your body into withdrawal, because it is now burning ketones instead of glucose for energy.

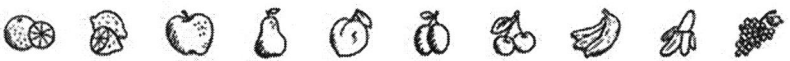

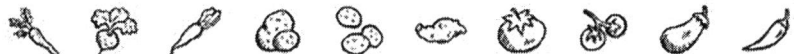

Symptoms differ from person to person, with varying degrees, but can include any of the following:

- ✓ Weakness
- ✓ Constipation
- ✓ Diarrhoea
- ✓ Headaches
- ✓ Nausea
- ✓ Irritability
- ✓ Dizziness
- ✓ Muscle cramps and / or soreness
- ✓ Vomiting
- ✓ Stomach pains
- ✓ Inability to concentrate
- ✓ Craving for sugar or sugary foods.
- ✓ Insomnia

Symptoms usually last for about a week, but can last longer for some people. It's important to know about keto flu and understand what's happening to you, so you don't give up, just as you're getting started. Fortunately, once you recognise that you have keto flu, there are ways to help you get through this miserable period.

1. **Stay hydrated:** Drink plenty of water.
2. **Don't overdo the exercise:** Your body is adapting itself to a new lifestyle, so why punish it even more with exercise? Yes, exercise is important, but during keto-flu, you need to rest.

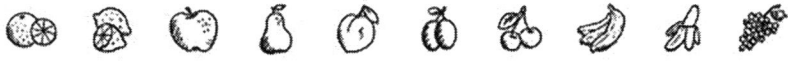

3. **Restore electrolytes:** The keto diet restricts food items that are high in things like potassium, and magnesium, so try to eat more green leafy veg or avos.

4. **Sleep:** The most common ailment experienced by new keto dieters, is fatigue, which results in irritability. Try limiting your caffeine, or have a warm bath with some lavender bath bombs.

5. **Eat plenty Fats:** Starting on the keto diet will result in cravings for naughty foods. But if you remain strict and eat enough fats, you will keep feeling satisfied and the cravings will disappear.

RECIPES

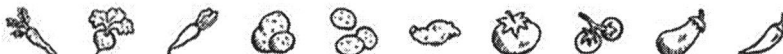

Breakfast

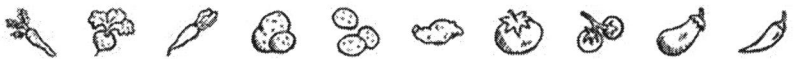

CHICKEN AND WAFFLE SANDWICHES

> *Serves: 4*
> *kCal: 421 | Carbs: 6.9g | Fat: 27.51g | Protein: 33.53g*

Ingredients

Waffles

- 2 tablespoons / 28.3g of melted butter
- 3 large eggs, separate the yolks and whites
- ¼ cup / 59ml of milk
- 1 cup / 130gr almond flour
- ½ teaspoon / 2½ gr of salt
- 1 teaspoon / 5ml of vanilla
- 1 tablespoon / 14gr of erythritol

Chicken

- 1 cup / 240ml of buttermilk
- 2 medium-sized chicken breast fillets
- 1 large egg
- 1 tablespoon / 14gr olive oil for frying
- Salt and pepper for taste
- 1 teaspoon / 5gr of paprika
- ¼ teaspoon / 2gr of cayenne powder

Directions

1. The night before, cut your chicken breast fillets in half, lengthwise. Cut them again, lengthwise, so you get 4 chicken strips. Soak them in the buttermilk overnight.
2. The following morning, season the soaked chicken with the salt, pepper, paprika and cayenne.
3. Preheat the oven to 350°F / 180°C and preheat your waffle maker.
4. In a mixing bowl, beat the 1 large egg.
5. In another mixing bowl, mix the almond flour with salt and pepper.
6. Place each chicken strip into the flour mixture, coating each side.

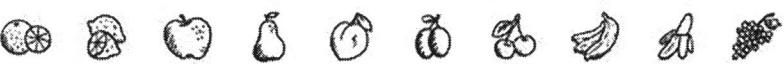

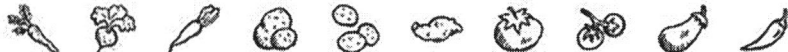

7. Now coat each chicken strip with the beaten egg, and the flour again, so there are two crumb layers.
8. Heat the olive oil in a skillet and quickly add the chicken, cooking each side of the chicken until they are browned.
9. Place the chicken strips onto a baking sheet, cover with some foil and bake in the oven for 15 minutes.
10. In another mixing bowl, whisk the egg yolks, erythritol, melted butter and vanilla together well.
11. Add the almond flour and some salt and whisk again until there are no more lumps.
12. With a hand mixer, beat the egg whites until they form stiff peaks.
13. Very carefully, adding a small portion at a time, fold the egg whites into the batter.
14. Spray some cooking spray on the waffle maker and add ⅓ cup / 79ml portions to it. Cook each waffle for about 5 to 6 minutes until browned.
15. Stack the waffle and chicken into a sandwich, keeping the pieces together with a toothpick, and serve.
16. You can add option extras like bacon or sugar-free syrup

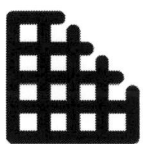

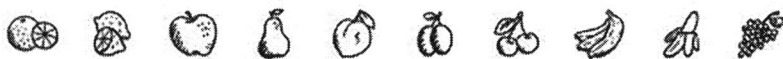

BREAKFAST BOWL

> Serves: 4
> kCal: 887.68 | Carbs: 8.2g | Fat: 75.4g | Protein: 40.95g

Ingredients

- 1 pound / 450gr of beef sirloin
- ¼ cup/ 59ml of soy sauce
- 2 tablespoons / 30ml of Calamansi juice*
- 6 medium-sized garlic cloves, minced
- 3 teaspoons/ 14gr of garlic powder
- 1 tablespoon / 14gr of granulated eythritol
- 1 cup / 128gr of coconut oil
- 1 pound / 455gr of cauliflower rice
- 4 large eggs
- Salt and pepper

Directions

1. In a mixing bowl, combine the soya sauce, Calamansi juice, garlic (leave some for later), garlic powder (leave some for later), erythritol, salt and pepper together. Mix until the salt and erythritol are completely dissolved.
2. Put the beef sirloin into a Ziploc bag and pour the marinade over the beef, in the bag. Seal the bag and place in the fridge overnight.
3. The following day, take the meat out of the bag.
4. Coat a frying pan with some of the coconut oil and heat. Add the beef to the pan and fry until all the liquid is almost absorbed. Turn the meat repeatedly.
5. Remove the beef and allow to cool, before slicing into strips.
6. Add the remaining coconut oil and minced garlic, garlic powder and some salt to the pan and sauté until it is aromatic.

*Calamansi juice is a Filipino variation of lemonade.

7. Toss in the cauliflower rice and coat evenly, cooking until the rice is tender
8. In a separate frying pan, fry the eggs as desired.
9. Once cooked, layer a bowl with the cauliflower rice, then the beef, top with the eggs and serve.

BLUEBERRY PANCAKE BITES

Serves: 6
kCal: 174.77 | Carbs: 7.07g | Fat: 13.27g | Protein: 6.52g

Ingredients

- 4 large eggs
- ¼ cup / 85gr of erythritol
- ½ teaspoon / 2½ ml of vanilla extract
- ½ cup / 170gr of coconut flour
- ¼ cup / 85gr of melted butter
- 1 teaspoon / 5gr of baking powder
- ½ teaspoon / 2½ gr of salt
- ¼ teaspoon / 2gr of cinnamon
- ⅓ cup / 80ml of water
- ½ cup / 170gr of frozen blueberries

Directions

1. Preheat the oven to 325°F/ 165°C.
2. Greaseproof a muffin tin extremely well, as the mixture is very sticky.
3. In a blender, mix the eggs, erythritol, and vanilla extract together.
4. To the mixture, add the coconut flour, melted butter, baking powder, salt and cinnamon and blend again, until smooth.
5. Allow the mixture to rest for a few minutes to thicken up.
6. Add the water in ▯ portions to the mixture, blending each time.
7. Blend until the mixture is scoopable, but not pourable.
8. Fill each muffin spot with the mixture, and top off with some blueberries, pushing them into the mixture.
9. Bake for 25 minutes. To test if they are ready, stick a toothpick into the center of one, and if it comes out clean, it's ready. If not, bake for a few mins more, checking all the time.
10. Serve with some sugar-free syrup.

STUFFED PEPPERS

> Serves: 4
> kCal: 245.5 | Carbs: 5.97g | Fat: 16.28g | Protein: 17.84g

Ingredients

- 4 large eggs
- 2 medium-sized bell peppers.
- ½ cup 170gr of ricotta cheese
- ½ cup / 170gr of shredded mozzarella
- ½ cup / 170gr of parmesan cheese, grated
- 1 teaspoon / 5gr of garlic powder
- ¼ teaspoon / 2gr of dried parsley
- ¼ cup / 85gr of baby spinach leaves
- 2 tablespoons / 28gr of extra parmesan cheese for garnishing

Directions

1. Preheat the oven to 375°F / 190°C.
2. Slice the peppers in equal halves and remove the seeds.
3. In a blender/food processor, add the cheeses, eggs, garlic powder and parsley and mix well.
4. Pour the mixture into each pepper half to just below the top. Add some spinach leaves and push them into the mixture with a fork.
5. Prepare a baking sheet, place the filled pepper halves onto the baking sheet and cover with foil.
6. Bake for about 35 – 45 minutes, or until the egg has set.
7. Sprinkle with the remaining parmesan cheese and grill for a further 3 – 5 minutes until the tops brown.

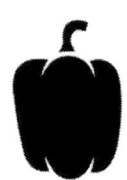

SPICY EGGS AND CHEESY HASH

> Serves: 3
> kCal: 248 | Carbs: 5.77g | Fat: 18.14g | Protein: 12.57g

Ingredients

- 5oz / 142gr of diced zucchini
- 6oz / 170gr of chopped cauliflower
- ½ medium-sized diced red bell-pepper
- 1 tablespoon / 15gr of melted coconut oil
- 1 teaspoon / 5gr of paprika
- 1 teaspoon / 5gr of onion powder
- ½ teaspoon / 2½ gr of garlic powder
- ¼ cup / 85gr of Mexican blend shredded cheese
- ½ of a medium-sized avocado, sliced
- 3 large eggs
- 3 tablespoons / 42gr of cotija cheese
- 2 teaspoons / 10gr of Tajin seasoning
- 1 tablespoon/ 5gr of sliced jalapeno (optional)

Directions

1. Preheat the oven to 400°F / 205°C.
2. Prepare a baking sheet with foil.
3. Spread in an even layer, the zucchini, cauliflower and red pepper and drizzle with the coconut oil.
4. Sprinkle on the veg, the onion powder, garlic and paprika and toss to coat everything well. Spread into a layer again.
5. Bake for around 10 – 15 mins until the veg begins to brown.
6. Take the veg out the oven and sprinkle the shredded Mexican cheese over the top.

7. Arrange the avo slices amongst the roasted veg and crack the 3 eggs into spaces in between.
8. Bake for a further 10 mins until the eggs are done.
9. Garnish with the cotija cheese, Tajin seasoning and optional jalapeno and serve.

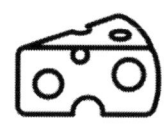

FAUX-TATOE BUBBLE AND SQUEAK

Serves: 3
kCal: 332.67 | Carbs: 8.6g | Fat: 28.11g | Protein: 10.65g

Ingredients

Mashed Cauliflower
- ½ of a medium-sized cauliflower, cut into florets
- 2 tablespoons / 28gr heavy whipping cream
- 1 tablespoon/ 15gr butter
- Salt and pepper to taste

Bubble and Squeak
- 3 bacon slices, diced
- 1 tablespoon/ 15gr of butter
- ¼ of a medium-sized onion, diced
- 1½oz / 50gr of leek, sliced
- 1 green onion, sliced
- 1½oz / 50gr of Brussels sprouts, chopped
- ¼ cup / 85gr of mozzarella
- ¼ cup / 85gr of parmesan cheese
- 2 tablespoons / 28gr of duck fat
- 1 teaspoon / 5gr minced garlic

Directions

1. A half of a medium-sized cauliflower is approximately 2 cups.
2. It's a good idea to prep all your veg beforehand, to make this go quicker.
3. Add your cauliflower florets, 1 portion of butter and the cream to a microwave-safe bowl and microwave on high for 4 minutes, uncovered. Mix well, once done.
4. Microwave for 4 minutes more, until the cauliflower is soft. Season with salt and pepper.
5. Using a stick blender, blend the cauliflower mixture until thick and creamy. While it's still hot, add the mozzarella so it melts. Set aside to cool down.

6. Using a pan on a medium-high heat, cook your bacon until crispy and the fat is rendered out.
7. Place the bacon on a paper towel.
8. Add the 2nd portion of butter to the bacon fat in the pan, along with the garlic, and cook for a minute on a medium heat.
9. Add the onion and cook until the onion is semi-transparent.
10. Add the leeks and Brussels sprouts and cook until soft. About 5 – 10 mins.
11. Add the green onion and cook for another minute.
12. Take off the heat and allow to cool.
13. Add the bacon to the veggie mix and then add the mashed cauliflower.
14. Taste and season if required.
15. Combine the veggies and mashed cauliflower well.
16. Using a separate pan, heated over a medium heat, add the duck fat.
17. Once it's melted, place egg rings into the pan and add some parmesan cheese inside the rings.
18. Add the cauliflower veggie mix to each ring and sprinkle some more parmesan over the top.
19. Warm each "pattie" through and flip, cooking until a crust forms.
20. Don't let them get too hot, as the mixture may run.

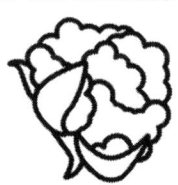

BACON BAGELS

Serves: 3
kCal: 605.67 | Carbs: 5.76g | Fat: 50.29g | Protein: 30.13g

Ingredients

Bagels
- ¾ cup / 98gr almond flour
- 1 teaspoon / 5gr xanthan gum
- 1 large egg
- 1½ cups / 510gr grated mozzarella cheese
- 2 tablespoons / 28gr cream cheese

Toppings
- 1 tablespoon / 15gr melted butter
- Some sesame seeds for taste

Fillings
- 2 tablespoons / 28gr pesto
- 2 tablespoons / 28gr cream cheese
- 1 cup / 340gr arugula leaves
- 6 slices of cooked bacon

Directions

1. Preheat the oven to 390°F / 200°C.
2. Mix together the almond flour and the xanthan gum.
3. Add the egg and mix until well combined, to look like a doughy ball.
4. Put a pot on a medium-low heat and slowly melt the cream cheese and mozzarella together. Take off the heat once melted.
5. Add the melted cheese mixture to the flour mixture and knead well. Persist through until is it well combined.
6. It's crucial that the xanthan gum is combined very well into the cheese mixture. If the dough gets tough, microwave for a few seconds to warm it and knead again until it resembles dough.

7. Divide the dough into 3 equal pieces and roll into logs.
8. Make the logs into circles by joining the ends together and place on a greased baking tray.
9. Melt the butter and brush the bagel tops and sprinkle on the sesame seeds.
10. Bake the bagels for around 18 minutes, until the tops are a golden brown. Keep an eye on them, as every oven is different.
11. Cook your bacon as desired.
12. Slice your bagels in half, spread some cream cheese, and add some pesto, arugula and bacon.

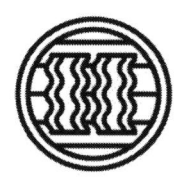

RICOTTA AND BLUEBERRY PANCAKES

> Serves: 5
> kCal: 311.4 | Carbs: 5.78g | Fat: 22.61g | Protein: 15.25g

Ingredients

- 3 large eggs
- ¾ cup / 200gr of ricotta cheese
- ½ teaspoon / 2½ gr of vanilla extract
- ¼ cup / 60ml of unsweetened vanilla almond milk
- 1 cup / 130gr of almond flour
- ½ cup / 65gr of golden flaxseed meal
- ¼ teaspoon / 2gr of salt
- 1 teaspoon / 5gr of baking powder
- ¼ teaspoon / 2gr of stevia
- ¼ cup / 85gr of blueberries

Directions

1. Preheat a skillet on a medium heat.
2. Blend the eggs, ricotta cheese, vanilla extract and almond milk together.
3. In a separate mixing bowl, mix the almond flour, flaxseed meal, salt, baking powder and stevia together.
4. Slowly add the dry Ingredients to the wet Ingredients and blend together until smooth.
5. Melt the butter in the skillet.
6. Using a 2 tablespoon measurement, scoop the batter and pour into the skillet.
7. Add 3-4 blueberries to each scoop/pancake.
8. When lightly browned on one side, flip and do the other side.
9. Serve with sugar-free syrup or extra berries

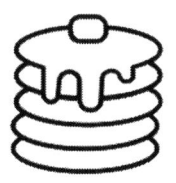

CHORIZO BAKED EGGS

Serves: 4
kCal: 321 | Carbs: 2.02g | Fat: 27.31g | Protein: 15.57g

Ingredients

- 5 large eggs
- 2oz / 56gr of Mexican-style pork chorizo
- 2 tablespoons / 28gr of butter
- Salt and pepper for tasting
- ⅔ cup / 85gr of shredded pepper jack cheese
- 1 medium-sized avocado
- 2 tablespoons / 28gr of sour cream
- 2 tablespoons / 28gr of chopped cilantro for some optional garnish

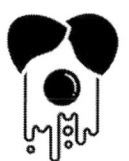

Directions

1. Preheat the oven to 400°F / 205°C.
2. Over a medium heat, preheat an oven-safe skillet.
3. Remove the chorizo casings and add the meat to the skillet. Fry until cooked and allow to drain on some paper towels.
4. Add the butter to the skillet and allow it to melt. Ensure the whole pan is evenly coated with butter. Take the pan off the heat and place on a heat-proof surface.
5. Into the buttered pan, crack 3 of the eggs and sprinkle with some salt and pepper.
6. Add some chorizo on top of the eggs and sprinkle cheese evenly over the whole dish.
7. Put the pan into the oven for 15 – 20 minutes, until you see the cheese start to bubble.
8. Bake for shorter periods if you prefer a more runny egg yolk.
9. Serve warm with the avo, sour cream and optional cilantro.

EGGS BENEDICT CASSEROLE

> Serves: 8
> kCal: 483 | Carbs: 2.78g | Fat: 33.41g | Protein: 18.54g

Ingredients

- 12 large eggs
- 8oz / 227gr of unsalted butter
- 19½oz / 553gr of peeled eggplant
- 1lb / 450gr of pre-cooked ham
- 6 large egg yolks
- ¼ cup / 60ml of heavy whipping cream
- Salt and pepper for tasting
- 2 tablespoons / 30ml of white vinegar
- ¼ teaspoon / 2gr of crushed peppercorns
- 1 tablespoon / 15gr of water
- Lemon juice for tasting

Directions

1. Preheat the oven to 375°F / 190°C.
2. Over a low heat in a heavy saucepan, melt your butter.
3. Once it's melted, you will notice foam rising to the surface. Remove this foam until it stops.
4. Carefully pour the melted butter into a heat-proof container, and prevent any solids from going with the butter.
5. Wash, chop and dice the eggplant.
6. Grease a casserole dish well and add the prepared eggplant.
7. Dice the ham and add it on top of the eggplant.
8. In a mixing bowl, crack the 12 eggs and season with some salt and pepper
9. Add the cream and whisk until well combined.
10. Pour the egg mixture over the ham and eggplant.
11. Mix around to make sure everything is well coated with egg mixture.
12. Cover the casserole with foil and bake for 30mins.
13. Uncover and bake for another 20 – 30 mins, until the egg is cooked.

14. While the casserole is in the oven, you can continue with the Hollandaise sauce.
15. Make sure your melted butter is still in liquid form and warm.
16. Preheat a skillet, add the vinegar and peppercorns and cook until the vinegar has almost evaporated. Add the water.
17. You will need a mixing bowl that can fit over a saucepan and be used as a double boiler.
18. Transfer the vinegar and peppercorn mixture to this mixing bowl.
19. Add the 6 egg yolks to the mixing bowl and whisk everything together.
20. Place the mixing bowl over a saucepan of boiling water.
21. Lower the heat and whisk until the egg yolks have thickened.
22. Remove from the heat and slowly drizzle the melted butter into egg yolk mixture, while whisking. Adding too quickly will break the emulsion, so go slowly.
23. Add the lemon juice and some salt to taste.
24. If your sauce requires thinning, add 2 – 3 tablespoons of water, one tablespoon at a time, until it reaches desired consistency.
25. Your casserole should be done by this point, so go ahead and pour the sauce over the casserole.
26. Garnish with whatever you like, such as green onion, or chives and serve.

EXCLUSIVE BONUS!

Get Keto Audiobook for FREE NOW!*

*The Ultimate Keto Diet Guide 2019-2020:
How to Loose weight with Quick and Easy Steps*

SCAN ME

or go to

www.free-keto.co.uk

*Listen free for 30 Days on Audible (for new members only)

Lunch

TUNA AND PESTO SALAD

Serves: 1
kCal: 604.8 | Carbs: 9g | Fat: 46.5g | Protein: 34.5g

Ingredients

Dressing
- 1 tablespoon / 15ml of olive oil
- ½ tablespoon / 7½ml of apple cider vinegar
- Salt and pepper for tasting

Salad
- 4 large iceberg lettuce leaves
- 1 small-sized tomato
- ½ of a small cucumber
- ¼ medium-sized avocado

Tuna
- 1 can of tuna in oil, drained
- 1½ tablespoons / 23gr of mayonnaise
- 1½ tablespoons / 23gr of full-fat Greek yogurt*
- 1 tablespoon / 15gr of pesto
- 2 teaspoons / 10ml of lemon juice
- Salt for tasting

Directions

1. Add the olive oil, vinegar, salt and pepper to a container with a secure lid. Close the lid and shake to combine everything together. Set aside.
2. Tear the lettuce leaves and place in a bowl.
3. Chop up the tomatoes, cucumber, and avo and add to the leaves.
4. In a separate bowl, mix the tuna, mayo, yogurt, pesto, lemon juice and some salt together.
5. Add the tuna mixture on top of the salad and drizzle with the dressing.

*You may want to substitute the yogurt for more mayo instead.

STEAK AND MUSHROOM STROGANOFF

Serves: 1
kCal: 594.52 | Carbs: 6.9g | Fat: 49g | Protein: 33.1g

Ingredients

- 1 tablespoon/ 15gr of butter
- Salt and pepper for tasting
- 4oz / 114gr of ribeye steak
- 4oz / 114gr of whole mushrooms, cut into quarters.
- 1 large garlic clove, minced
- 3 tablespoons / 45ml of chicken stock
- 1½ oz / 43gr of cream cheese
- ¼ teaspoon / 2ml of Worcestershire sauce
- ¼ teaspoon/ 2gr of black pepper (for the sauce)
- 1 teaspoon / 5gr of minced parsley

Directions

1. Over a medium-high heat, preheat a skillet and add half of the butter.
2. Add the steak to the pan, sprinkle some salt and pepper over the steak and sear it. Set aside.
3. Add the remaining butter to the pan and once melted, add the mushrooms and cook until they have softened.
4. Lower the heat to low, add the garlic and cook for another minute.
5. Add the chicken stock, and using a wooden spoon, scrape the brown bits from the bottom of the pan. This is all the flavour!
6. Add the cream cheese, Worcestershire sauce, black pepper and stir together until the cheese has melted.
7. Put the steak on a plate, top it off with the stroganoff sauce, garnish with the parsley and serve.

CHEESY BEER SOUP

> Serves: 6
> kCal: 382.82 | Carbs: 6.87g | Fat: 30.3g | Protein: 17.39g

Ingredients

- 3 cups / 705ml of chicken stock
- 1 bottle (12oz)/ 350ml low carb beer
- ½ cup / 120ml heavy whipping cream
- 2 teaspoons / 10gr of xanthan gum
- 6 slices of cooked and diced bacon
- 12oz / 341gr of grated cheddar cheese
- 1 tablespoon / 15gr of butter
- ½ cup / 130gr of diced onion
- 2 cloves of minced garlic
- ½ of a small red bell-pepper, diced
- 1 tablespoon / 15ml of Dijon mustard
- 1 teaspoon / 5gr of celery salt
- 1 teaspoon / 5gr of black pepper
- ½ teaspoon / 2½ gr of paprika
- ¼ teaspoon / 2gr of cayenne pepper

Directions

1. Get out your stock pot and heat it over a medium heat.
2. Add the butter and heat it up.
3. Once it's hot, add the bell-pepper and onion and sauté until they have softened.
4. Add the garlic and cook until the garlic is aromatic.
5. Pour in the beer, chicken stock and the heavy cream.
6. Add the celery salt, black pepper, paprika and cayenne pepper, stirring occasionally while it heats up.
7. Adding the xanthan gum may start clumping so to prevent that, add a little of the soup to a small bowl. Add the xanathan gum to this and whisk together. Then add that to the main pot of soup.

8. Continue stirring until the soup thickens

9. A handful at a time, add the cheese. Allow it to dissolve before adding the next handful.

10. Pour into serving bowls, add the diced bacon on top and serve.

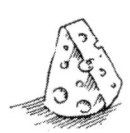

SALMON BURGERS ON CEDAR PLANK

> *Serves: 4*
> *kCal: 360.25 | Carbs: 1.7g | Fat: 16.76g | Protein: 47.08g*

Ingredients

- 1½lb / 680gr freshly caught salmon filets
- 1½ tablespoons / 45gr of mayonnaise
- 1½ tablespoons / 45gr of mustard
- ½ of a small red onion, diced
- 2 tablespoons / 28gr of fresh dill
- 1 celery stalk, diced
- 2 minced garlic cloves
- 2 teaspoons / 10gr of salt
- 1 teaspoon / 5gr of black pepper
- Fresh lemon juice for tasting

Directions

1. You will require some cedar planks that you can find in many grocery stores in the grilling section. They give amazing flavor to your food, so why not give it a go?
2. Soak your cedar planks in water, for 2 hours before you start cooking. Make sure you get enough planks for all your salmon burgers.
3. Preheat the grill (indirect heat), to around 350°F / 180°C.
4. Prepare your salmon by removing the skin and any bones.
5. Cut into small pieces and add to a food processor.
6. Add the mayonnaise, mustard, dill, salt, pepper and the garlic on top of the salmon.
7. Pulse the food processor until the salmon becomes like a smooth paste.
8. Put everything into a mixing bowl and add the onion and celery.
9. Put the soaked planks onto the grill and allow them to warm up.
10. Form the salmon mixture into burger shapes.
11. Place two burgers on each plank and grill them for about 20 – 35 minutes until the salmon is cooked through.

12. Take the planks off the heat, and squeeze some lemon juice on top of the burgers.

13. Serve with your favorite toppings.

BACON CHEESEBURGER KEBABS

> Serves: 10
> kCal: 303.41 | Carbs: 3.29g | Fat: 23.4g | Protein: 18.45g

Ingredients

Kebabs

- 1lb / 455gr of ground beef
- 1 tablespoon/ 15ml of Worcestershire sauce
- ½ teaspoon / 2½gr of salt
- 1 teaspoon / 5gr of black pepper
- 1 teaspoon/ 15gr of dried minced onion
- 6 slices of bacon
- 5 slices of cheddar cheese, cut into quarters
- ½ a head of an iceberg lettuce
- 10 cherry tomatoes
- 20 dill pickle slices

Dipping Sauce

- ½ cup / 120ml mayonnaise
- 2 tablespoons/ 30ml of sugar-free ketchup
- 1 tablespoon/ 15ml of mustard
- 2 tablespoons/ 28gr of minced onion
- 2 tablespoons/ 28gr of minced dill pickles
- Pickle juice for tasting

Directions

1. Preheat the grill at 375°F / 190°C. You will need to be able to do direct and indirect grilling.
2. In a mixing bowl, add the ground beef, Worcestershire sauce, salt, pepper, garlic powder, and dried minced onion and mix together well.
3. Scoop out and form evenly sized balls.
4. Flatten them out into a burger shape.
5. Place a cast iron skillet over the indirect heat and cook the bacon. Not too crispy, as you still need to put it on the skewer. Once cooked, set aside.

6. Place the skillet back onto the indirect heat and add your burger patties. Cook one side, turn and cook until cooked through.
7. Move the skillet to the direct heat and sear both sides of the burgers.
8. Once cooked through, add a slice of cheese to the top of the burgers, and allow to melt. Set aside.
9. Using large skewers stack the patties, bacon, lettuce, tomatoes, and pickle slices.
10. Mix the dipping sauce Ingredients together in a bowl and serve with the kebabs.

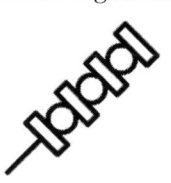

TACO-STUFFED AVOS

Serves: 1
kCal: 392.17 | Carbs: 6.3g | Fat: 46.49g | Protein: 13.23g

Ingredients

For the Filling

- 7oz / 198gr of cauliflower
- 1 cup / 120gr of raw walnuts
- 1 tablespoon/ 15gr of hulled hemp seeds
- 1 teaspoon/ 5gr of cumin
- 1 teaspoon/ 5gr of garlic powder
- 1 teaspoon/ 5gr of onion powder
- 2 teaspoons/ 10gr of smoked paprika
- 2 teaspoons / 10gr of adobo sauce
- 4 tablespoons / 60ml of avocado oil, divided between 2 tablespoons
- 2 tablespoons / 10gr of grated cheddar
- 1 teaspoon / 5gr of salt

For the Avocado Boats

- ½ cup / 170gr of taco filling
- ½ of a medium-sized avocado
- 1 tablespoon of sour cream
- 1 tablespoon of grated cheddar

Directions

1. Divide the cauliflower up into florets and add to a food processor.
2. Add the walnuts, hemp seeds and seasonings to the food processor.
3. Pulse until the cauliflower and nuts become like a crumble.
4. Heat one half of the avocado oil in a skillet, over a medium heat.
5. Add one half of the "taco meat" (cauliflower) mixture to the skillet, stir well until the nuts are toasted and the cauliflower softens
6. Add half the adobo sauce to the skillet, folding it into the mixture. Make sure the mixture is browning evenly.

7. Take off from the heat and fold in the cheese, season with salt and put into a bowl.
8. Repeat with the rest of the taco filling.
9. Slice the avo in half, remove the stone.
10. Scoop a portion of the avo out to make room for the taco filling.
11. Fill the avo with ½ cup of your prepared taco mixture, top with sour cream and cheddar.

BACON SALAD WITH KALE

> Serves: 2
> kCal: 328.55 | Carbs: 6.23g | Fat: 27.85g | Protein: 13.5g

Ingredients

- 4 slices of bacon
- 2 cups / 134gr of kale
- ¼ cup / 35gr of sweet onion
- ½ cup / 60gr of raw walnuts
- 2 teaspoons / 6gr of erythritol
- ½ teaspoon / 2½ ml of maple syrup
- 1 tablespoon / 15ml of lemon juice

Directions

1. Cook the bacon to the desired crispiness.
2. Place bacon on a plate and allow to cool.
3. Add the walnuts to the bacon grease in the pan and cook on a medium heat, stirring enough to coat all the nuts.
4. Cut the kale leaves into bite-sizes and remove the stems. Put into a bowl.
5. Dice the onion.
6. Sprinkle the erythritol and maple syrup over the walnuts in the pan. Stir to coat evenly.
7. Add the onion to the walnuts and sauté until soft and the walnuts have caramelized.
8. Take the pan off the heat and drizzle some lemon juice over the top.
9. Cut the bacon strips into smaller bits.
10. Pour the maple walnut mixture over the kale and toss to coat evenly.
11. Sprinkle the bacon over the top and serve.

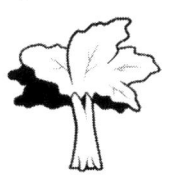

EGGS BENEDICT SALAD WITH BACON

Serves: 3
kCal: 333.63 | Carbs: 2.5g | Fat: 31.73g | Protein: 14.77g

Ingredients

- 3 strips of bacon
- 3 tablespoons / 27gr of grated parmesan cheese
- 3 cups / 550gr of spring mix greens
- 6 halved cherry tomatoes
- 2 medium egg yolks
- ¼ cup / 55gr of butter
- 1 teaspoon / 5ml of lemon juice
- 3 medium eggs, poached
- 1 tablespoon / 0.45gr of dried chives

Directions

1. Cook bacon to desired crispiness, drain and cool.
2. Lightly spray some non-stick spray onto a microwave safe plate. To the plate add the parmesan cheese in 3 separate mounds. Microwave until the mounds are crispy. Take out the microwave and allow to cool.
3. Add the egg yolks and lemon juice to a blender and blend until the mixture is a pale yellow.
4. Microwave the butter until it starts to bubble. Add this melted butter to the blender mixture and blend until combined. Should be light in color and thicken as it cools.
5. Put the greens, tomatoes and bacon slices on to a plate.
6. Add a layer of parmesan cheese on top.
7. Add the poached eggs on top of the cheese and pour your hollandaise sauce over them.
8. Garnish with chives.

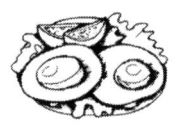

PRESSED HALLOUMI WITH BLACKBERRY, BASIL AND SPINACH

Serves: 1
kCal: 434 | Carbs: 5.7g | Fat: 32.3g | Protein: 27.6g

Ingredients

- 4oz / 115gr of halloumi cheese
- 2 teaspoons/ 9½gr of mayonnaise
- ¼ cup / 45gr of spinach
- 4 leaves of basil, torn
- 0.8oz / 23gr of sliced cucumber
- 6 whole blackberries, sliced in half

Directions

1. Warm up your Panini press to a medium heat.
2. Slice the halloumi into equal-sized rectangles.
3. Put the halloumi on the Panini press and cook until it starts to brown.
4. Flip the halloumi and brown the other sides.
5. On one of the halloumi slices, Layer the mayo, spinach, cucumber, basil, and blackberries.
6. Take the other halloumi slice and place it on top of the fillings to make a sandwich.
7. Close the press and hold for one minute.
8. Switch off the press.
9. Plate the halloumi sandwich, top with any remaining berries and serve warm.

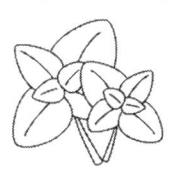

Dinner

IN-A-SKILLET PHILLY CHEESESTEAK

> Serves: 5
> kCal: 535.74 | Carbs: 8.72g | Fat: .35.64g | Protein: 42.74g

Ingredients

- 1 tablespoon / 15ml of olive oil
- 1 medium-sized onion, cut in half
- 2 teaspoons / 10gr of mince garlic
- 1 cup / 250gr of green bell-pepper, diced
- 1lb / 455gr of ground beef
- 1 teaspoon / 5gr of salt
- ¼ teaspoon / 2gr of black pepper
- ¼ teaspoon / 2gr of garlic powder
- ¼ teaspoon / 2gr of onion powder
- ½ cup / 120ml of beef broth
- 1b / 455gr of cauliflower florets
- 8oz / 227gr of sliced mushrooms
- ¼ cup of half and half
- 10 slices of provolone cheese

Directions

1. Dice one half of the onion and thinly slice the other half.
2. In a large skillet, add the olive oil. Once it's heated, add half of the onion, the garlic, and half of the bell-pepper. Sauté until the veggies begin to soften.
3. Add the ground beef and season it with the onion powder, garlic powder, salt and half of the black pepper. Crumble the beef with a potato masher.
4. Cover the skillet and cook for a few more mins, stirring now and then until the beef is completely cooked.
5. Add the beef broth, cauliflower, onions, bell-pepper and mushrooms and stir. Allow to simmer for 15 mins and then mash the cauliflower into smaller pieces.
6. Turn off the heat and stir in the half and half.
7. Season with the remaining pepper, onion and garlic powders.
8. Spread the cheese slices over the top and cover with a lid.
9. Cook until the cheese has melted.

INSTANT POT FAUX-LASAGNA

Serves: 8
kCal: 403.24 | Carbs: 7.36g | Fat: 26.85g | Protein: 30.9g

Ingredients

- 1lb / 450gr of ground beef
- 2 cloves of minced garlic
- 1 small diced onion
- 1½ cup / 340gr of ricotta cheese
- ½ cup / 70gr of parmesan cheese
- 2 large eggs
- 25oz / 740ml of marinara sauce
- 8oz / 230gr of sliced mozzarella cheese
- 1 cup / 235ml of water

Directions

1. Set your Instant Pot to the sauté setting and brown the beef, garlic and onion.
2. In a mixing bowl, mix the ricotta, parmesan and eggs together well.
3. Switch off the Instant Pot, remove the beef and drain the grease.
4. Add the marinara to the beef and mix well. Leave some sauce for the top of the dish.
5. Take out a spring-form pan and wrap the base with foil. The spring-form pan must be able to fit in to the Instant Pot.
6. On the spring-form pan, layer your meat, mozzarella cheese and ricotta, until everything is in the pan.
7. Top off with the left over marinara sauce.
8. Over the pan loosely with some foil.
9. Add the cup of water to the Instant Pot, then the rack and then the spring-form pan onto the rack.
10. Close the Instant Pot lid and valve and cook on a high pressure for 9 minutes.
11. Release the valve and serve.

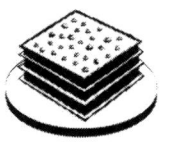

CHICKEN SALAD WITH BACON

> Serves: 4
> kCal: 725.12 | Carbs: 5.38g | Fat: 57.29g | Protein: 37.86g

Ingredients

- 2 tablespoons / 24gr of olive oil
- 1.1oz / 500gr of chicken breast filets, cut into cubes
- 1 clove of minced garlic
- 5 slices of chopped bacon
- 1 cup / 65gr of sliced mushrooms
- ⅓ cup / 43gr of fresh basil
- 5oz / 140gr of fresh spinach
- 3 – 4 small-sized sun-dried tomatoes
- 1 cup / 235ml of sugar-free ranch dressing

Directions

1. Put a frying pan over a medium heat and add the olive oil.
2. Once the oil is hot, add the chicken cubes and brown them.
3. Just before the chicken is done, add the garlic and mix well. Cook until the chicken is done.
4. Take the chicken out of the pan and put into a mixing bowl. Set aside.
5. Add bacon to the same pan and cook until it's reached your desired crispiness. Once done, add to the chicken.
6. Add the mushrooms, basil and some of the spinach to the chicken and bacon and mix until the spinach wilts.
7. Put the remaining spinach into a serving bowl and spread the chicken mix over the top.
8. Garnish with the tomatoes and ranch dressing.

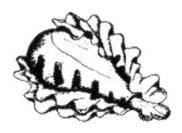

SALISBURY STEAK AND CAULI MASH

> Serves: 3
> kCal: 512.07 | Carbs: 6.77g | Fat: 35.83g | Protein: 37.23g

Ingredients

- 3 cups / 700gr of cauliflower florets
- 1 tablespoon / 15gr of butter
- 3 tablespoons / 45ml of almond milk (preferably unsweetened)
- 12oz / 340gr ground beef
- ¼ cup / 32gr of almond flour
- 2 teaspoons / 2gr of chopped fresh parsley
- 2 teaspoons / 10ml of Worcestershire sauce
- ¼ teaspoon / 2gr of onion powder
- ¼ teaspoon / 2gr of garlic powder
- Salt and pepper for tasting
- 1 tablespoon / 15ml of olive oil
- 1½ cup / 100gr of sliced mushrooms
- ¼ cup / 60ml of beef broth
- 2 tablespoons / 15gr of sour cream

Directions

1. Preheat the oven to 375°F / 190°C and line a baking sheet with foil.
2. Boil a pot of water, liberally seasoning with salt. Add the cauliflower and boil until tender.
3. Drain the cauliflower and put it into a mixing bowl. Add the butter and almond milk and mash it up.
4. In a separate mixing bowl, mix the beef, flour, Worcester sauce, onion powder, garlic powder, salt, pepper and parsley together well.
5. Divide the beef mixture into burger patties shapes to create your "steaks" and place them on the lined baking sheet. Bake until the "steaks" are cooked through.
6. Place a large skillet over a medium-high heat and add the olive oil.
7. Add the mushrooms and cook until they are brown and tender.

8. Add the beef broth, stirring often, scraping the bits forming on the bottom.
9. Add the sour cream and whisk to combine. Season with some salt and pepper
10. Serve the "Salisbury Steaks" on top of the cauli mash and top it off with the mushroom sauce.

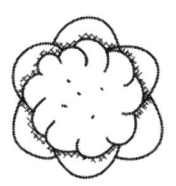

FAUX CRAB CAKES

Serves: 3
kCal: 434.24 | Carbs: 5.47g | Fat: 41.01g | Protein: 10.03g

Ingredients

- 1 can of hearts of palm. Drain the liquid.
- 2 tablespoons / 30ml of mayonnaise
- 1 teaspoon / 5gr of Old Bay seasoning
- 1 tablespoon / 1gr of parsley
- ¼ cup / 32gr of almond flour
- 1 large beaten egg
- 1 tablespoon / 10gr of diced onion
- 1 teaspoon / 5gr of butter
- 3 tablespoons / 42gr of almond meal
- 2 tablespoons / 18gr of parmesan cheese
- 4 tablespoons / 60ml of avocado oil

Directions

1. Shred the hearts of palm with a fork, until it resembles crab meat.
2. Add the Old Bay seasoning, mayo, almond flour, egg and parsley and mix until combined.
3. Heat the butter over a medium heat in a skillet, and sauté the diced onion until it's translucent. Gently fold the onions into the hearts of palm "crab meat".
4. In a shallow bowl, mix together the almond meal and parmesan for a coating.
5. Separate the "crab meat" into 6 equal balls and press into the coating, squashing the balls into cakes. Make sure the cakes are completely covered.
6. Heat a skillet over a medium-high heat and add the avocado oil.
7. Fry each cake, turning carefully to brown each side. Preferably fry two at a time.
8. Serve hot.

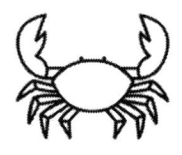

MUSHROOM STEAKS WITH AVO SALSA

Serves: 2
kCal: 328.8 | Carbs: 5.45g | Fat: 29.95g | Protein: 5.45g

Ingredients

For the Marinade

- 2 tablespoons / 30ml of avocado oil
- 1 tablespoon / 15ml of liquid aminos
- 1 teaspoon / 5ml of liquid smoke
- 2 cloves of minced garlic
- ½ teaspoon / 5gr of cumin
- 1 teaspoon / 5ml of balsamic vinegar

For the Mushrooms

- 2 large Portobello mushroom caps
- 1 medium-sized diced avocado
- ½ of a medium-sized roma tomato, diced
- ½ cup / 20gr of finely minced parlsey
- 2 tablespoons / 28gr of hulled hemp seeds
- ½ teaspoon / 2.5gr of salt

Directions

1. In a small mixing bowl, whisk all the marinade Ingredients together.
2. Clean and trim the mushrooms, including the stem if desired.
3. Using a shallow dish, soak the mushrooms with the marinade and ensure they are completely coated. Let them rest in the marinade, turning occasionally, for about 5 minutes.
4. In a separate mixing bowl, combine the avocado, tomato and parsley. Sprinkle some salt and half of the hemp seeds over this. Toss to evenly coat.
5. Preheat a skillet over a medium-high heat and pan sear the mushrooms, until each side is browed and the mushrooms are tender.
6. Top each mushroom with the avo salsa and residual hemp seeds and serve.

CREAMY SPINACH ALFREDO WITH ZUCCHINI CURLS

Serves: 5
kCal: 420.82 | Carbs: 7.12g | Fat: 36.7g | Protein: 16.42g

Ingredients

- 2 medium-sized zucchini
- 1½ cups / 375gr of ricotta
- 1 cup / 235gr of parmesan cheese. Divide in half.
- 2 teaspoons / 1gr of dried basil
- 1 medium-sized egg
- 4 tablespoons / 57gr of butter
- 2 medium-sized cloves of garlic, minced
- 1 cup / 950ml heavy cream
- ½ cup / 30gr baby spinach, chopped roughly
- ½ oz / 7gr of sun-dried tomatoes

Directions

1. Preheat your oven to 350°F / 180°C.
2. Spray non-stick spray over a casserole dish.
3. Slice each zucchini lengthwise with a wide vegetable peeler to make "ribbons". You will need about 20 "ribbons" to fill a small casserole dish.
4. In a large mixing bowl, add the ricotta, half of the parmesan, basil, spinach and egg and mix well. Place in a large freezer bag and set aside for later. This bag will be used as a piping bag, so make sure it's adequate. (Use a piping bag if you have one)
5. In a saucepan, heat the butter, garlic and cream over a medium heat. Add the remaining parmesan and stir until the sauce has thickened. Take off from the heat.
6. Pour a third of the sauce into the bottom of the casserole dish.
7. Secure the top of the freezer bag / piping bag and cut the tip as if you're going to pipe some frosting. Squeeze / pipe the mixture over the zucchini "ribbons".
8. Roll each strip gently, so as not to squeeze the filling out.
9. Place each zucchini curl sideways into the sauce in the casserole dish.

10. Add the sundried tomatoes to the remaining sauce and stir.
11. Pour the sauce over the zucchini curl.
12. Cover the dish with some foil and bake for 25 – 30 mins until the top of the sauce is browned and bubbling.
13. Take out the oven, allow to cool slightly and serve.

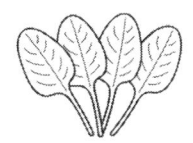

CHICKEN MEATLOAF CUPCAKES

> *Serves: 6*
> *kCal: 316.568 | Carbs: 2.72g | Fat: 23.87g | Protein: 24.82g*

Ingredients

Buffalo Gravy

- 1½ tablespoons / 21gr of unsalted butter
- 1 medium-sized minced garlic clove
- ⅔ cup / 150gr of wing sauce
- 1 teaspoon / 5ml of Worcestershire sauce
- 1½ tablespoons / 22ml of white vinegar
- Salt and pepper for tasting

For the Chicken

- 1 tablespoon / 15ml of extra-virgin olive oil
- ½ a medium-sized diced onion
- ½ cup / 50gr of minced celery
- 1lb / 455gr of ground chicken
- 1 teaspoon / 5ml of Worcester sauce
- 2 medium-sized minced garlic cloves
- ½ cup / 110gr of crushed pork rinds
- Salt and pepper for tasting
- 1 large egg
- 2 tablespoons / 30ml of chicken broth
- ½ teaspoon / 2.3gr of unflavored gelatin
- ¼ teaspoon / 0.54gr of celery seed
- 2oz / 55gr blue cheese
- 2½ tablespoons / 36gr of unsalted butter

Directions

1. Preheat your oven to 375°F / 190°C.
2. Over a low heat, melt the gravy butter in a saucepan.

3. Add the 1 garlic and cook for a minute. Add the wing sauce, Worcestershire sauce, vinegar, salt and pepper to the garlic and whisk to combine. Simmer for a minute and set aside.
4. In a skillet over a medium heat, warm the olive oil, add the onion, celery and 2 garlic. Cook until soft and set aside to cool down.
5. In a mixing bowl, whisk the egg and chicken broth together. Add the gelatin and allow to bloom for 5 mins.
6. In the bowl with the onion mixture, add the chicken, Worcestershire sauce, celery seed, pork rinds, salt, pepper and a quarter of the prepared wing sauce. Add the whisked egg and mix to combine.
7. Spray a cupcake tin with some non-stick spray and add about 2 tablespoons of the mixture to each cupcake spot. Using your finger, make a space in the center of each one and add blue cheese and a slice of butter. Top each one with the remaining meat mixture and brush some wing sauce over the lid.
8. Put it in the oven and bake for 25 minutes, brushing more sauce on top every 10 minutes.

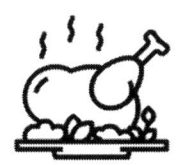

SHRIMP AND CAULIRICE

Serves: 4
kCal: 315.05 | Carbs: 5.89g | Fat: 25.23g | Protein: 17.43g

Ingredients

For the Caulirice
- 1 teaspoon / 5gr of coconut oil
- ½ cup / 110gr of coconut flakes, unsweetened
- 2 cups / 480gr of cauliflower florets

For the Shrimp
- 1 teaspoon / 5gr of coconut oil
- ¼ of a medium-sized diced sweet onion
- 2 medium-sized minced garlic cloves
- 1¼ cups / 300ml of canned coconut milk
- 24 medium-sized tail on precooked shrimp, frozen
- 3 sprigs of chopped cilantro
- ½ of a medium-sized lime, juiced
- 2 tablespoons / 28gr of crushed red pepper

Directions

1. Warm up a non-stick skillet for the caulirice.
2. Heat the coconut oil and sauté the coconut flakes until slightly brown.
3. Add the cauliflower florets to a food processor / blender and pulse until it looks like rice.
4. Add the caulirice to the skillet and stir.
5. Sauté until the coconut is toasted and the caulirice is softened
6. Don't be tempted to add extra liquid, just let it fry in the coconut oil.
7. Take the caulirice and coconut out of the skillet and place in a covered container until ready for serving.

8. In the same skillet, add the coconut oil, garlic and onion and sauté until aromatic.
9. Add in the coconut milk and stir until it simmers
10. Allow it to reduce for 5 mins.
11. Add the shrimp to the coconut sauce and cook on a medium-low heat until the shrimp is tender and begins to curl.
12. Add the lime juice and cilantro and gently stir.
13. Dust the red pepper over the shrimp.
14. Dish up the caulirice, layer the shrimp on top and drizzle with sauce.

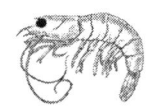

Desserts and Snacks

COCONUT AVOCADO SMOOTHIE

> Serves: 4
> kCal: 252.75 | Carbs: 3.7g | Fat: 26.25g | Protein: 2.68g

Ingredients

- 1 medium-sized avocado, cut in half
- 14oz / 400gr can of coconut milk
- 2½ tablespoons / 25gr of allulose
- 2oz / 60ml of water
- 8oz / 227gr of ice cubes
- ¼ tablespoon / 5½gr of vanilla bean extract

Directions

1. If you notice that the coconut milk has separate, just whisk together until it's fully incorporated.
2. Using a blender or a smoothie maker, add the avocado halves, coconut milk, allulose, water, ice and vanilla.
3. Blend until thick and smooth.
4. Pour into a glass and serve. You can top it off with some whipped coconut cream or grilled coconut cubes to make it more decadent.
5. This smoothie is a great option for fat boosting your keto diet

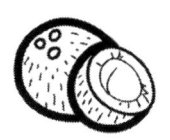

NEAPOLITAN CHIA DESSERT

Serves: 3
kCal: 187.07 | Carbs: 4.53g | Fat: 11.47g | Protein: 6.27g

Ingredients

- ½ cup / 81gr of chia seeds
- 1½ cups / 355ml of unsweetened almond milk
- 2 tablespoons / 28gr of monk fruit sweetener
- 1 teaspoon / 5ml of vanilla extract
- 4 medium-sized diced strawberries
- 2 teaspoons / 10gr of unsweetened cocoa powder

Directions

1. In a mixing bowl, mix the chia seeds, almond milk, sweetener and vanilla together. Leave to chill in the fridge for 10 – 15 mins until firm.
2. Take out the fridge and divide equally between three bowls.
3. To one of the bowls, add the cocoa powder and mix. Taste and add more sweetener if required.
4. Cook the strawberries in the microwave for 30 seconds until soft and mash with a fork.
5. Mix the mashed strawberries into another chia seed bowl.
6. You will now have one bowl of chocolate, one bowl of strawberry and one bowl of vanilla, which will form your layers.
7. In small glasses, layer each one repeatedly. You can even lay some sliced strawberries against the sides of the glass, as you layer up.

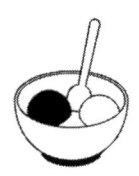

ALMOND AND COCONUT COOKIES

Serves: 12
kCal: 58.92 | Carbs: 0.83g | Fat: 5.01g | Protein: 2.31g

Ingredients

- 2 large egg whites
- 8 tablespoons / 114gr of allulose
- 1 cup / 70gr of sliced almonds
- ¼ cup / 55gr of unsweetened coconut flakes

Directions

1. Set your oven to 325°F / 162°C
2. Line some baking sheets with baking paper.
3. In a mixing bowl, combine the egg whites and the allulose.
4. Add the sweetener and whisk until the mixture thick. Must not be foamy.
5. Add the sliced almonds and coconut flakes and stir until combined.
6. Whip mixture until it resembles a cookie batter.
7. Scoop the batter into mound and place on the lined baking sheet, spacing the mounds evenly.
8. Flatten the mounds to form cookies.
9. Bake for 10 mins and turn the baking sheet around to get an even bake.
10. Bake for a further 8 mins until the cookies are toasted and crispy.
11. Take out and leave to cool.

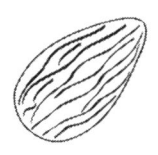

COCONUT AVO ICE CREAM

> Serves: 8
> kCal: 222.38 | Carbs: 6.88g | Fat: 21.09g | Protein: 2.07g

Ingredients

- 1 medium-sized avocado
- 1 can of coconut milk
- ½ cup / 120ml of heavy cream
- ¾ cup / 96gr of allulose
- 1 medium-sized lime
- 1 cup / 220gr of coconut flakes

Directions

1. Cut the avo, remove the stone and scoop out the avo insides. Add it to a blender.
2. Along with the avo, add the coconut milk, cream, and allulose and blend until smooth.
3. Take the line and juice and zest it. Add the juice and zest to the blender and blend again for a minute.
4. Place in the fridge for a minimum of an hour.
5. Add the coconut flakes to a warm pan and toast until lightly brown around the edges. Take off the heat.
6. Take out your ice cream machine and add the chilled avo mixture to it. Churn according to the machines' Directions.
7. Place it in a freezer safe container and freeze.
8. When ready to serve, garnish with some coconut flakes.

COCOCHOC MUG CAKE

> Serves: 2
> kCal: 219 | Carbs: 2.95g | Fat: 19.06g | Protein: 7.23g

Ingredients

- 2 tablespoons / 14gr of coconut flour
- 2 tablespoons / 15gr of cocoa powder
- 2 tablespoons / 15gr of Swerve confectioners (or erythritol)
- ¼ teaspoon / 2gr of baking powder
- 2 large eggs
- 2 tablespoons / 30gr of melted butter
- 2 tablespoons / 30ml of unsweetened almond milk

Directions

1. Mix together the coconut flour, cocoa powder, sweetener and baking powder.
2. Add the eggs, butter, and almond milk and mix well.
3. Grease a large coffee mug and pour in the cake batter.
4. Place in the center of your microwave and cook for 2 minutes. Keep an eye, as every microwave is different. When you see the cake popping over the top of the mug, it's done.
5. Carefully take out of the microwave as it can be hot.
6. Remove from the mug, slice in half and serve.

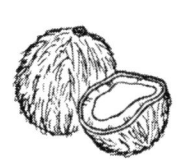

14 Day Meal Plan

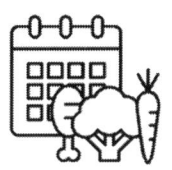

*indicates a new meal not mentioned previously in this book

DAY 1

Breakfast*: Coconut and Berry Oatmeal

Calories: 445 | Carbohydrates: 6.34g | Fat: 38.16g | Protein: 10.45g

Ingredients

- 2 tablespoons / 28gr of ground flaxseed
- 1 tablespoon / 14gr of almond meal
- 1 tablespoon / 14gr of desiccated coconut
- ½ teaspoon / 2½gr of vanilla powder
- ½ teaspoon / 2½gr of cinnamon
- ⅓ cup / 80ml of coconut milk
- ½ cup / 120ml of almond milk
- ¼ cup / 85gr of mixed berries
- 1 teaspoon / 5gr of dried pumpkin seeds

Directions

1. Place a saucepan on the stove to preheat it.
2. Add everything except the berries and pumpkin seeds to the saucepan.
3. Stir continuously until the mixture is hot and thick like oatmeal
4. Pour the mixture into a bowl, add the berries and seeds and serve.

Lunch: Steak and Mushroom Stroganoff (see page 54)

Dinner: Chicken Salad with Bacon (see page 69)

DAY 2

Breakfast: Breakfast Bowl (see page 37)

Lunch*: Casserole Sub Sandwich

Calories: 312.43 | Carbohydrates: 3.12 g | Fat: 22.11g | Protein: 24.91g

Ingredients

- 8oz / 227gr of smoked deli ham slices
- 8 slices of swiss cheese
- 16 slices of dill pickles
- 3 tablespoons / 45ml of Italian dressing
- ¼ tablespoon / 7½ ml of Italian seasoning

Directions

1. Preheat the oven to 375°F / 190°C
2. In a casserole dish, spread out the ham slices in a layer.
3. Add a layer of swiss cheese on top of the ham.
4. Add the dill pickles, dressing and seasoning.
5. Bake for 10 – 15 minutes until the cheese has melted

Dinner: Faux Crab Cakes (see page 72)

DAY 3

Breakfast: Blueberry Pancake Bites (see page 39)

Lunch: Bacon Salad with Kale (see page 63)

Dinner*: Cheese and Broccoli Soup

Calories: 418.85 | Carbohydrates: 5.62g Fat | 38.68g | Protein: 12.45g

Ingredients

- 1 tablespoon / 15gr of butter
- 1 small-sized onion, chopped
- 2 medium-sized cloves of garlic, minced
- Salt and pepper for tasting
- ½ teaspoon / 2½gr of xanthan gum
- ½ cup / 120ml of chicken broth
- 1 cup / 184gr of broccoli, chopped
- 1 cup / 240ml of heavy cream
- 1½ cup / 180gr of grated cheddar cheese

Directions

1. Preheat a pot on a medium heat.
2. Add the butter, onions, garlic, salt and pepper to the pot and sauté until the onions are see-through
3. Sprinkle the xanthan gum over the onions mixture.
4. Pour in the chicken broth and stir.
5. Add the broccoli to the pot and make sure the broth coats all the veg.
6. Add the cream and stir quickly and frequently, ensuring the xanthan gum gets mixed in and thickens. Bring to a boil.
7. Add the cheese and slowly whisk until all has melted.
8. Dish into soup bowls, garnish with broccoli and cheese and serve.

DAY 4

Breakfast*: Cheese and Mushroom Omelette

Calories: 515 | Carbohydrates: 4.17 g | Fat: 39.58g | Protein: 21.34g

Ingredients

- 3 large eggs
- 2 teaspoons / 10ml of heavy cream
- 3oz/ 85gr of mushrooms, sliced
- 1 teaspoon / 5ml of olive oil
- 2oz / 56gr of crumbled goats cheese
- Some Spike seasoning for taste
- Optional green onions for garnishing

Directions

1. Heat the oil in a frying pan and fry the mushrooms until soft.
2. Whisk together the eggs, heavy cream and some Spike seasoning.
3. Remove the mushrooms from the pan and set aside.
4. Add the egg mixture to the pan and cook for 2 to 3 minutes.
5. When you see the egg starting to set, add the cooked mushrooms and goats cheese.
6. Carefully fold the omelette over and cook until the goats cheese begins melting.
7. Serve and garnish with green onions, if desired.

Lunch: Bacon Cheeseburger Kebabs (see page 59)

Dinner: Salisbury Steak and Cauli Mash (see page 70)

DAY 5

Breakfast: Spicy Eggs and Cheesy Hash (see page 41)

Lunch*: Avo Bowls

Calories: 169.13 | Carbohydrates: 2.53g | Fat: 14.52g | Protein: 3.27g

Ingredients

- 3 medium-sized avocados, chopped in half, stones removed
- 1½oz / 50gr of chopped mushrooms
- 1 medium-sized chopped green onion
- 10 chopped cherry tomatoes
- 1oz / 44gr of crumbled goats cheese
- 1 tablespoon / 15ml of olive oil
- 1 tablespoon / 15ml of liquid smoke
- ½ teaspoon / 2½gr of paprika
- 3 tablespoons / 45ml of balsamic vinegar

Directions

1. Place a frying pan over a medium heat to warm.
2. In a mixing bowl, add the mushrooms, onions and tomatoes.
3. In the warmed pan, heat the olive oil, liquid smoke and paprika.
4. Add the goats cheese to the pan, and sauté until the cheese has browned.
5. Take the pan off the stove and add the goats cheese to the mixing bowl. Mix together.
6. Scoop out a portion of the avo halves to make room for the filling.
7. Spoon the mixture into the holes in the avos. Garnish with the scooped portion of avo.
8. Pour a ½ teaspoon of balsamic vinegar onto each and serve.

Dinner: Shrimp and Caulirice (see page 78)

DAY 6

Breakfast: Chorizo Baked Eggs (see page 48)

Lunch: Steak and Mushroom Stroganoff (see page 54)

Dinner*: Creamy Chicken

Calories: 382.79 | Carbohydrates: 4.33g | Fat: 25.93g | Protein: 31.85g

Ingredients

- 2 slices of chopped bacon
- 2lb / 910gr of chicken breast filets (boneless and skinless)
- 16oz / 450gr of cream cheese
- ½ cup / 120ml of water
- 2 tablespoons/ 30ml of apple cider vinegar
- 1 tablespoon / 0.45gr of dried chives
- 1½ teaspoon / 5gr onion powder
- 1½ teaspoon / 5gr garlic powder
- 1 teaspoon / 2½gr of crushed red pepper flakes
- 1 teaspoon / 2½gr of dried dill
- Salt and pepper for tasting
- 2oz / 55gr of grated cheddar cheese
- 1 medium-sized sliced green onion

Directions

1. Set your Instant Pot to the sauté and allow to heat up. Add the bacon and cook until its crisp. Take the bacon out and set aside, hitting cancel on your Instant Pot.
2. Add the chicken, cream cheese, water, vinegar, chives, garlic powder, onion powder, red pepper flakes, dill, salt and pepper to the Instant Pot.
3. Manually set it to high pressure for 15 minutes. Once done, do a quick release.
4. Remove the chicken and shred it. When done, return it to the pot.
5. Add in the cheddar and stir.
6. Dish up the mixture, sprinkle the bacon and green onions on top and serve.

DAY 7

Breakfast: Breakfast Bowl (see page 37)

Lunch*: Taco Salad

Calories: 388.37 | Carbohydrates: 6.5g | Fat: 32.47g | Protein: 15.8g

Ingredients

- ¾lb / 340gr of ground beef
- 1 teaspoon / 5gr of ground cumin
- ½ teaspoon / 1.3gr of chili powder
- 1 teaspoon / ½gr of dried parsley
- 1 teaspoon / 3gr of garlic powder
- 8oz / 227gr of chopped romaine lettuce
- 9oz / 255gr of chopped iceberg lettuce
- 2 small chopped red tomatoes
- 1½ cups / 180gr of grated mozzarella cheese
- 1 medium-sized chopped avocado
- 1 cup / 120gr of sour cream

Directions

1. Place the ground beef into a non-stick pan.
2. Add the herbs and spices to the beef and cook on a medium heat.
3. Once done, take off the heat and allow the beef to drain and cool. Set aside for later.
4. In a salad bowl, add the chopped lettuce, tomatoes, mozzarella and avocado and mix well.
5. Add the ground beef and sour cream on top of the salad mix and serve.

Dinner: Mushroom Steaks with Avo Salsa (see page 73)

DAY 8

Breakfast: Eggs Benedict Casserole (see page 49)

Lunch: Salmon Burgers on Cedar Plank (see page 57)

Dinner*: Chicken Cordon Bleu Soup

Calories: 580.17 | Carbohydrates: 3.93g | Fat: 50.74g | Protein: 27.43g

Ingredients

- 6 small bacon strips
- 2 cups / 470ml of heavy whipping cream
- 6oz / 170gr of cream cheese
- 1 tablespoon / 14gr of butter
- 2 cups / 470ml of chicken stock
- 2 cups/ 200gr of grated Swiss cheese
- 1 cup / 150gr of ham, cubed
- 6oz / 170gr of chicken breast, shredded
- 2 cups / 134gr of chopped kale with stems removed

Directions

1. Over a medium-low heat, fry the bacon until crispy. Roughly chop it and set aside. Reserve about ¼ of the bacon for the garnish.
2. To a large soup pot, add the heavy cream, butter and cream cheese and heat over a medium heat. Cook until everything has melted.
3. Add the chicken stock to the soup pot and bring to a simmer.
4. Add the grated cheese and stir until completely melted.
5. Add the ham, chicken and ¾ of the bacon, mix and simmer.
6. Add the kale, stir and cook without the lid for 10mins, until the kale begins to soften.
7. Garnish with the bacon and serve hot.

DAY 9

Breakfast*: Breakfast Egg Wraps

> Calories: 412 | Carbohydrates: 2.26 | Fat: 31.66 | Protein: 28.21

Ingredients

- 10 large eggs
- Salt
- Pepper
- 1½ cups / 510gr of grated cheddar
- 5 slices of cooked bacon
- 5 patties of cooked breakfast sausage

Directions

1. Preheat a non-stick skillet on a medium-high heat.
2. Take 2 of the eggs and whisk.
3. Lower the heat to a medium-low, once the skillet is hot and add the whisked eggs.
4. Greaseproof a muffin tin extremely well, as the mixture is very sticky.
5. Season with some salt and pepper.
6. Cover the skillet with a lid and allow the egg to cook almost all the way through.
7. Sprinkle some cheese over the egg.
8. Add a strip of bacon and half of a sausage patty on the egg.
9. Carefully roll the egg over the fillings like a wrap. Take it slow, as it can be tricky.
10. Set aside.
11. Repeat all the steps for the next 4 egg wraps and serve.

Lunch: Tuna and Pesto Salad (see page 53)

Dinner: In-A-Skillet Philly Cheesesteak (see page 67)

DAY 10

Breakfast: Stuffed Peppers (see page 171)

Lunch*: Zucchini Salad

Calories: 206.4 | Carbohydrates: 4.33g | Fat: 14.59g | Protein: 11.55g

Ingredients

- 2 medium-sized zucchinis
- 8 slices of cooked bacon
- 1 cup / 200gr of feta cheese, cubed
- 1 cup / 200gr of chopped cherry tomatoes
- 4 tablespoons / 60ml of balsamic vinegar

Directions

1. Slice the zucchinis into ribbons using a grater or a peeler.
2. In a salad bowl, add the zucchini ribbons and top off with the tomatoes, bacon and cheese.
3. Drizzle with the vinegar and toss before serving.

Dinner: Faux Crab Cakes (see page 72)

DAY 11

Breakfast: Ricotta and Blueberry Pancakes (see page 47)

Lunch: Cheesy Beer Soup (see page 55)

Dinner*: Cauli Casserole

Calories: 537.53 | Carbohydrates: 8.21g | Fat: 42.73g | Protein: 31.12g

Ingredients

- 1 small-sized cauliflower
- 1 cup / 230gr of cream cheese
- 1 cup / 230gr of grated cheddar cheese
- 4 sliced of chopped bacon
- ¼ cup / 100gr of chopped mushrooms
- 1 medium-sized chopped jalapeno
- 2 medium-sized boneless, skinless, chicken thighs

Directions

1. Preheat your oven to 350°F / 180°C.
2. Chop the cauliflower into florets and add to a casserole dish.
3. In a mixing bowl, add the cream cheese, cheddar, jalapeno, mushrooms and bacon and mix well.
4. Add the cheese mixture to the cauliflower and mix well.
5. Lay the chicken on the cauliflower mixture and mix gently.
6. Bake for one hour, until the cheese has melted and the chicken has cooked.

DAY 12

Breakfast*: Pizza Eggs

Calories: 333 | Carbohydrates: 4.28g | Fat: 22.66g | Protein: 25.59g

Ingredients

- 3 large eggs, separated
- 4 tablespoons / 57gr of grated mozzarella cheese
- 1 teaspoon / 5gr of Italian herb blend
- 2 large sliced black olives
- 4 large mild pepper rings
- 1 tablespoon / 15gr of diced red bell-pepper
- 1 tablespoon / 15gr of tomato sauce (preferably Rao's)

Directions

1. You will need 2 microwave-safe ramekin-sized bowls
2. Add 1 tablespoon of the mozzarella cheese and Italian herb seasoning to each bowl.
3. In a mixing bowl, beat the egg whites until just frothy, and pour into the bowls.
4. Microwave for 1-2 minutes until the whites are cooked. Allow to cool.
5. Beat the egg yolks and scramble lightly in a frying pan.
6. Fold the pizza toppings into the scrambled egg yolks and take off the heat.
7. Add some tomato sauce to your cooked egg white "pizza bases".
8. Add the scrambled egg mixture and remaining cheese on top of the tomato sauce.
9. Cook for another 20 seconds in the microwave, until the cheese has melted.
10. Serve hot.

Lunch: Taco-Stuffed Avos (see page 61)

Dinner: Chicken Salad with Bacon (see page 69)

DAY 13

Breakfast: Bacon Bagels (see page 45)

Lunch*: Vegan Scrambled No-Eggs

Calories: 211.4 | Carbohydrates: 4.74g | Fat: 17.56g | Protein: 10.09g

Ingredients

- 14oz / 400gr of firm tofu
- 2 tablespoons / 28gr of diced yellow onion
- 3 tablespoons / 45ml of avocado oil
- 1½ tablespoons / 22½gr of nutritional yeast
- ½ teaspoon / 2½gr of garlic powder
- ½ teaspoon / 2½gr of turmeric
- ½ teaspoon / 2½gr of salt
- 1 cup / 340gr of baby spinach
- 3 diced grape tomatoes
- 3oz / 85gr of vegan cheddar

Directions

1. You need to gently squeeze out some of the water in the tofu, so wrap it in some paper towels or a clean cloth and squeeze.
2. On a medium heat, place a skillet and sauté the onion and a third of the avo oil, until the onion is soft.
3. Add the tofu to the skillet and using a potato masher or a fork, crumble the tofu, until it resembles scrambled egg.
4. Drizzle the remaining avo oil over the tofu.
5. Sprinkle the tofu with the dry seasoning and stir to coat evenly.
6. Cook over a medium heat, stirring and folding until most of the liquid has gone.
7. Fold in the spinach, tomato and cheese and cook until the cheese has melted and the spinach has wilted.

8. Serve hot.
9. Leftovers can be stored in your fridge for 3 days.

Dinner: Chicken Meatloaf Cupcakes (see page 76)

DAY 14

Breakfast: Chicken and Waffle Sandwiches (see page 35)

Lunch: Pressed Halloumi with Blackberry, Basil and Spinach (see page 35)

Dinner*: Roast Chicken in Red pepper Gravy

Calories: 156 | Carbohydrates: 0% (1.2g) | Fat: 15% (10g) | Protein: 24% (12g)

Ingredients

Chicken Thighs

- 1½lb / 680gr of chicken thighs, boneless and skinless
- Salt and pepper for tasting
- 1 tablespoon / 15gr of coconut oil
- 4oz / 113gr of goats cheese
- 2 tablespoons / 5gr of chopped fresh parsley

Roasted Red Pepper Gravy

- 4oz / 113gr of roasted red peppers
- 2 garlic cloves
- 2 tablespoons / 30ml of olive oil
- ½ cup / 120ml of heavy cream

Directions

1. Warm up your oven to 350°F / 180°C and place a skillet on a medium-high heat.
2. Season the chicken with salt and pepper.
3. Put the coconut oil in the skillet to melt. Once melted, add the chicken and sear for 5 mins on each side, until browned.
4. Add the red peppers, garlic and olive oil to a blender and puree everything. Add the heavy cream and blend again until thoroughly combined.
5. Take the skillet off the heat and pour the gravy over the chicken. Flip the chicken and coat evenly in the gravy.

6. Sprinkle the goats cheese over the chicken.
7. Place the skillet in the oven to bake the chicken for 10-15 minutes.
8. Garnish with some fresh parsley and serve.

5 Quick Tips to Losing Weight with Keto

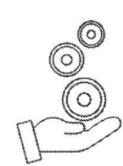

1. **Set realistic goals for yourself:** Reading stories of other peoples' keto successes can be inspiring, but you don't see the struggles they experience getting to their successes. Also, every person responds differently to keto, and you have to find that balance within the diet that works for you. It's important to not compare yourself to others, so you avoid getting discouraged. So, with keto, you need to be more realistic with yourself and your goals, rather than overly strict.

2. **Take it slowly:** Losing quickly makes you feel great, but it's also not sustainable or healthy for you. Realistically, you should be aiming for 2lb / 1kg of weight loss per week. And don't climb on the scales too often either! Keep a record of a weekly weigh in and waist measurement and if you think it's going too slowly, change up the diet.

3. **Keep it Simple:** If you want to try your hand at the keto diet, keep it simple. Just keep reminding yourself that it's High-Fat and Low-Carb and you will see results.

4. **Eating out:** Just because you're on diet, doesn't mean you have to forego that birthday at a restaurant. Choose a meal that has meat or fish and change up the fries for extra veg. Have a burger without the buns. For dessert have a bowl of berries with some fresh cream.

5. **Clean out your Closet:** By that we mean your kitchen cupboard. Keeping treats in the kitchen will create temptations. While some days you will have the strength to say no, there will be days when you are not so motivated, and knowing that candy bar is in the back of the cupboard, will gnaw at you.

EXCLUSIVE BONUS!
Get Keto Audiobook for FREE NOW!*

*The Ultimate Keto Diet Guide 2019-2020:
How to Loose weight with Quick and Easy Steps*

SCAN ME

or go to

www.free-keto.co.uk

*Listen free for 30 Days on Audible (for new members only)

Low Carb

Introduction

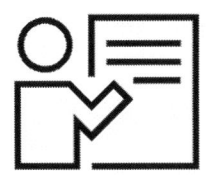

Chances are, you've heard the term "low carb" at some point. In fact, lately, it's become one of the diet buzzwords that everyone seems to be talking about. However, have you ever wondered what it really means? Let's take a look:

What is Low Carb?

Carbs- such as flour and white sugar- while they may taste great, can result in a variety of health issues, including sugar imbalances. However, you can kickstart your body's' metabolism by decreasing the amount of carbs you consume. This encourages your body to burn excess fat for energy.

When you consume carbs, they are converted into glucose, which will remain provide your body with a quick energy boost. If not used right away, your body will store the glycogen in your liver and muscles to be used later. If you consume excess carbs that your body really doesn't need, they are converted into fat. Later, when you consume more carbs, your body uses those instead of tapping into your fat stores. You may not know it, but if your diet is rich in carbs, your body will just keep using those- and storing what it doesn't need at the moment. This causes your body's natural fat-burning process to shut down.

The worst part about it is, since your body easily digests carbs, they don't really do much to stop hunger pangs. Therefore, shortly after you eat a meal high in carbs, you'll be hungry again- craving more carbs. Proteins and fats take longer to digest, which means you don't get as hungry as often. Additionally, when you decrease your consumption of "bad" carbs, your glucose levels stabilize, so your energy levels stay pretty stable instead of spiking and dipping all the time. When your blood sugar levels are stable, your body doesn't produce as much insulin (aka, the "fat storage" hormone), which also means you don't experience as many hunger pangs.

Unfortunately, most diets are really only beneficial in the short term and are difficult to maintain because you are restricting your fat and calories, which means you feel hungry all the time. However, when done properly, a low-carb diet is a great approach to eating. In fact, some individuals have reported improvements in medical conditions such as PCOS, epilepsy, and diabetes. Of course, please don't just take our word for it. If you have been diagnosed with a serious medical condition, you should speak with your physician before making any significant changes to your diet.

History of Low Carb

While it's true that low carb diets are really just making headlines, many people have depended upon them for some time due to their health and weight loss benefits. In fact, William Banting, a British undertaker in the Victorian Era who was obese, spoke with several medical specialists to try to get some help with weight loss. Eventually, an ear specialist suggested a radical diet that would limit his consumption of carbs, especially things such as sugar, butter, bread, milk, and potatoes (which were dietary staples of that time). This new way of eating helped him lose a lot of weight, as well as helped give him some relief from many of the ailments that accompanied his obesity.

Now that you have some of the history behind the low-carb way of life, let's look at some things you need to know about carbs.

Everything You Need to Know About Carbs

The very first thing you need to know is this: what is a carbohydrate? A carbohydrate is any large group of starches, cellulose/gums, and sugars that are alike because they are made up of oxygen, hydrogen, and carbon in similar quantities. Your body uses carbs by processing them and turning them into glucose, which is a simple sugar, to fuel it. Typically, 1 g carb is 4 calories.

Now that you know what is meant by the term "carb", you need to know more about what foods contain carbs. You will find simple carbs/simple sugars in refined/processed sugars such as honey, candy, and table sugar- in addition to fruits, veggies, and milk products. Your body will have an easier time digesting simple carbs over complex carbs.

On the other hand, a complex carb is a long chain of simple carbs and are made of starch and fiber. Foods that contain complex carbs encompass starchy veggies- such as potatoes, bread, pasta, cereals, and rice.

You're probably wondering now if that means that some carbs are better/healthier than others. The truth is, when you start a low-carb diet, it's ideal to eliminate them from your diet. However, since complex carbs contain other nutrients, they are better for you than simple carbs. Still, when comparing sugars based on their health value, an apple isn't any better than honey or table sugar. Regardless of the source, your body processes sugar the exact same way.

According to nutritionists, around 55-60% of your daily caloric intake should be from carbs. That's right, when eaten in moderation, carbs are really not all that bad for you. One FDA report revealed what when you consume sugar in moderate quantities, it can't be linked to dependency or any medical conditions. Of course, if you consume too much sugar, you may develop cavities and become obese. However, scientists have not linked sugar to hyperactivity and, in fact, have suggested that sugar may actually be calming for both adults and children.

What Happens in Our Body?

As you've learned, most carbs are made up of large chains of sugar molecules. Before these chains can be absorbed into your blood and used, your body must break them down through the process of digestion.

This process begins in your mouth, where salivary amylase enzymes break down starches (the sugars that exist in potatoes and grains) into smaller molecules. After that, carbs go through your stomach basically unchanged and into your small intestine. At that point, the enzymes in your small intestine will convert the carbs into simple sugars (glucose & fructose). Then, the sugars can go into your bloodstream and be used by your body. They will either be: used for fuel, saved for later, or stored as fat.

Used for Fuel

When it comes to energy, carbs are the body's primary source. Sure, it's true that your body can use fat and protein as energy- after the carb portion of your meal has been burned. Carbs travel through your bloodstream in the form of fructose and glucose and your bodily tissues absorb them. Your body is able to freely absorb fructose- but needs insulin to absorb glucose. The insulin drives the glucose into your muscles so that they can contract. Once the glucose and fructose have absorbed into your cells, they combine with oxygen to create adenosine triphosphate (ATP)- which is the currency your cells use for energy.

Saved for Later

Once your energy requirements have been met, the remaining carbs will travel to your muscles and liver. At that point, the body will convert it into glycogen, which is a long chain of glucose molecules. Glycogen is a stored form of energy that your body can use to meet energy requirements between your meals or when you're fasting. Your body uses glycogen to balance your glucose levels and help you avoid experiencing hypoglycemia.

Stored as Fat

According to the experts, about 500 grams of glycogen is stored in your muscles and liver. This is equal to 2,000 calories, which can meet the energy requirements of your body for around 18 hours. Any carbs that are not needed for this glycogen storage will then be converted into fatty acids, which your body stores in fat cells as triglycerides. The triglycerides are a concentrated energy source- but your body will only burn them once the glycogen has been depleted. This mechanism was evolved by the human body to protect us against long fasting periods. However, in modern society, fasting/depriving your body of calories is typically done on purpose- known as dieting.

Is Low Carb Really Healthy?

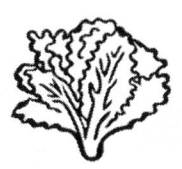

For many years, low carb diets have been the subject of controversy. Some people hold the belief that low-carb diets actually cause your cholesterol to increase and could lead to heart disease. After all, they do typically encourage high fat consumption. The scientific community has actually proven that low-carb diets/lifestyles are actually quite beneficial and healthy. Experts say that low-carb diets will encourage weight loss and improve risk factors for heart disease.

In this section, we're going to explore a few of the health benefits of low-carb diets.

Decrease Overall Appetite

One of the worst side effects of dieting is hunger and is one of the primary reasons that most people are miserable and end up giving up on their diet. Experts say that low-carb dieting automatically reduces your overall appetite because when people cut carbs and increase their consumption of fat and protein, they are not eating nearly as many calories.

More Weight Loss at First

One of the most effective- and simplest- ways to drop a few pounds is to cut carbs. Studies have proven that individuals who go reduce their carb consumption will actually lose weight quickly than those who reduce fact consumption, even though individuals on low fat diets restricting the number of calories they consume.

This is because a low-carb diet actually gets rid of the water weight, which decreases your insulin levels and causes you to lose weight quickly at first. There are some studies that indicate that those who restrict their carb consumption will lose 2-3 times as much weight- and don't' feel like they're starving themselves.

One particular study showed that a low carb diet was especially effective for the first six months when compared with conventional weight loss methods. However, after that, there wasn't a significant difference between the various methods.

More Fat is Lost from Abdomen Area

One thing you need to know is that the fat in your body is not all the same. The way it affects your overall health and risk factors for various medical conditions depends on where it is stored in your body. Fat is categorized into two main types:

- Subcutaneous: under the skin
- Visceral: abdominal area

Visceral fat typically is found surrounding your organs. This type of fat has been associated with inflammation and insulin resistance and could be the driving force behind metabolic dysfunction.

Experts are quick to point out that most people who lose weight on a low carb diet seem to lose it from their abdominal area. Eventually, this could result in a decreased risk of heart disease and type 2 diabetes.

Drastic Reduction in Triglycerides

Triglycerides are the fat molecules that circulate through your bloodstream. Experts have determined that high triglyceride levels after an overnight fast increase your risk of heart disease. Sedentary individuals typically have high triglyceride levels because of their carb consumption.

However, when you start cutting carbs, you're likely to experience a significant reduction in triglycerides in your blood. However, if you consume a low-fat diet, you are more likely to experience the opposite: an increase in triglycerides in the blood.

"Good" HDL Cholesterol Increases

HDL, or high-density lipoprotein- cholesterol is often referred to as "good" cholesterol. The higher your HDL compared to LDL ("bad" cholesterol), the lower your risk of heart disease. One way to increase your HDL cholesterol levels is to consume fat- which is a major component of low-carb diets. Therefore, it's obvious that your HDL will increase on a low-carb diet, while it will only slightly increase or possibly decline on a low-fat diet.

"Bad" LDL Cholesterol Decreases

In addition to increasing your HDL, a low-carb diet also decreases your LDL cholesterol. LDL is known as "bad" cholesterol and contributes to heart disease. Individuals who have elevated LDL levels are more likely to experience a heart attack.

Experts say that in this case, size matters, small LDL particles indicate an increased risk of heart disease, while large ones indicate a decreased risk. The low-carb way of life will decrease the number of LDL particles in your blood and make them bigger.

Therefore, since decreasing your carb consumption increases HDL and decreases LDL, it's actually a great diet for your overall heart health.

Reduction in Insulin and Blood Sugar Levels

Some experts say that low-carb diets are beneficial for those who have insulin resistance and diabetes, which affects millions of people across the world. Studies have revealed that cutting carbs drastically decreases insulin and blood sugar levels. In fact, some individuals with diabetes have claimed that after beginning a low-carb diet, they were able to decrease their insulin dosage by half. In one study of individuals with type 2 diabetes showed that those who started a low-carb diet were able to eliminate (or at least decrease) their medication within 6 months.

Of course, if your physician has prescribed medication to regulate your blood sugar, you'll need to discuss any changes in your diet with him/her. You may need to make adjustments to your medication to avoid hypoglycemia.

Decrease Blood Pressure

One risk factor for several medical conditions is high blood pressure/hypertension. According to the experts, a low carb diet is quite effective for lowering blood pressure, which will decrease your risk of these- and therefore, lead to a longer life.

Treats Several Brain Disorders

Some areas of your brain are powered only by glucose, which is the reason your liver produces it from protein when you're limiting/eliminating carbs from your diet. However, much of your brain also burns ketones, which your body produces during periods of starvation or when you are limiting carbs. This is the point of the ketogenic diet. Professionals have used it for years to treat children with epilepsy that have not responded to medication.

There are many cases in which children on this diet have been cured of epilepsy. One study showed children on this carb-limiting diet had a 50% reduction in the number of seizures they experienced, and 16% of them experienced no seizures. Medical experts are considering low-carb diets as a treatment for other brain conditions, such as Parkinson's and Alzheimer's.

What it comes down to is this: there are very few things that have as many health benefits as the low-carb diet. This lifestyle will have many positive impacts on your overall health, such as:

- Decreasing your appetite

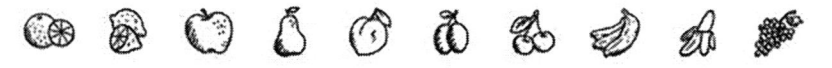

- Lowering triglycerides
- Increase weight loss
- Improved blood sugar, cholesterol, and blood pressure

If you believe that this type of diet is a good idea for you, make sure that you take the time to speak with your physician before taking drastic measures.

What Should I Avoid?

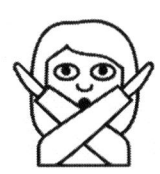

When you set out on a low carb eating plan, it's obvious that foods such as candy, cakes, and sugary sweet drinks should be avoided. However, when it comes to figuring out which staple foods you need to be limiting or avoiding, it can be a bit more challenging. The truth is that some of these are actually healthy, just not great for those on a low-carb eating plan.

Your target daily carb count will determine whether you should completely eliminate these foods or just limit them. Typically, a low carb diet consists of 20 to 100 grams of carbs daily. Following, you'll find 14 foods that you should avoid (or at least limit) when you get started on your low carb diet.

Breads/Grains

Bread comes in a variety of forms, such as tortillas, bagels, rolls, loaves, and flatbreads- and in many cultures, is a staple food. Unfortunately, they're all high in carbs- whether they are made from refined flour or whole-grains. While it's true that the actual carb count will depend upon the portion sizes and ingredients, following are the average carb counts for breads:

- 1 slice white bread: 14 g carbs/1 g is fiber
- 1 slice whole wheat bread: 17 g carbs/2 g is fiber
- 10-in flour tortilla: 36 g carbs/2 g is fiber
- 3-in bagel: 29 g carbs/1 g is fiber

As you can see, depending upon your limits, eating a sandwich, bagel, or burrito could cause you to reach- if not exceed it. In addition, most grains including oats, wheat, and rice have high carb counts and must be limited or avoided on a low carb diet.

Some Fruits

One important fact to note is that eating lots of fruits and veggies has proven to decrease an individual's risk of heart disease and some cancers. On the other hand, many fruits have lots of carbs and are not great for the low-carb dieter. Please note: a typical serving of fruit is 1 cup/120 grams or 1 small piece. For example, one small apple contains 21 g carbs, 4 g are from fiber. Therefore, if you're on a low carb diet, it's probably best to avoid some fruits, especially those that are really sweet and dried, which have higher carb counts.

Following are a few fruits with their carb counts:

- 1 medium banana: 27 g carbs/3 g from fiber
- 1 oz/28 g raisins: 22 g carbs/1 g from fiber
- 2 large dates: 36 g carbs/4 g from fiber
- 1 cup/165 g sliced mango: 28 g carbs/3 g from fiber
- 1 medium pear: 28 g carbs/6 g from fiber

On the other hand, berries have more fiber and less sugar than most other fruits, so- even on a low carb diet- you can enjoy them in moderation (1/2 cup, or 50 grams).

Starchy Veggies

Most diets- even low carb ones- do allow you to have an unlimited consumption of low starch veggies. After all, most veggies are high fiber, which can help maximize weight loss and balance glucose levels. On the other hand, there are some veggies that are high starch that contain less fiber and more carbs, and therefore should be limited on low carb diets.

If you're trying to stick to a very low carb diet, it's best to avoid the following completely:

- 1 cup/175 g corn: 41 g carbs/5 g from fiber

- 1 medium potato: 37 g carbs/4 g from fiber

- 1 medium sweet potato/yam: 24 g carbs/4 g from fiber

- 1 cup/150 g cooked beets: 16 g carbs/4 g from fiber

Again, most low carb diets do allow you to have lots of low carb veggies.

Pasta

Pasta is versatile and cheap- so it's great for those who are on a budget. However, it's very high in carbs, so it's not ideal for those who are on a low carb diet. In fact, 1 cup/250 grams of pasta has 43 grams carbs- and only 3 of those are from fiber. Don't assume that whole wheat pasta is much better: one serving has 37 grams of carbs- and only 6 grams are from fiber.

Therefore, if you're on a low carb diet, spaghetti or other pasta isn't really the best idea unless you eat a smaller portion- which, truthfully, is not easy for most people. If you really can't give up your pasta, consider trying some shirataki noodles or spiralizing some veggies instead (zucchini makes great noodles).

Breakfast Cereal

We all know that the sugary breakfast cereals are full of carbs- but are you aware that even the so-called "healthy" options have high carb counts too? For example, 1 cup/90 grams of cooked oatmeal contains 32 grams carbs, only 4 from fiber.

Even steel cut oats, which are considered healthier, because they're not as processed as most other forms of oatmeal are not a great option: ½ cup/45 grams contains 29 grams carbs, 5 from fiber.

The whole grain cereals are even worse: a ½ cup/61 gram serving of granola contains 37 grams carbs, 7 from fiber. The same serving size of Grape Nuts contains 46 grams carbs, 5 from fiber.

Therefore, it's best to avoid (or at least minimize) breakfast cereals when you're on a low-carb diet because one serving could very easily throw you over the limit- before you even add the milk.

Beer

Even if you're on a low carb diet, you don't have to completely give up alcohol. You can still enjoy it in moderation. After all, hard liquor contains zero carbs and dry wines have very few. However, beer is actually full of carbs. In fact, one 12-oz/356 ml can contains 12 grams of carbs- and even light beers contain 6 grams per can.

Some experts caution that liquid carbs actually cause weight gain more than carbs from solid foods because they're not as filling and don't really satiate your appetite as much as food does. Therefore, if you still want to enjoy alcohol from time to time on your low carb diet, try spirits or dry wines.

Sweetened Yogurt

Yogurt is both versatile and tasty. While it's true that plain yogurt typically has a fairly low carb count, most people prefer to enjoy fruity, sweet nonfat/low-fat varieties. Unfortunately, these sweetened varieties contain high carb counts.

In fact, 1 cup/245 grams of sweetened, nonfat fruit yogurt typically has around 47 grams carbs, much higher than a serving of ice cream the same size. However, if you choose ½ cup/123 grams of plain Greek yogurt with ½ cup/50 grams of raspberries or blackberries will keep the carb count less than 10 grams.

Juice

When you commit to a low carb diet, juices are a terrible idea. While it's true that it provides you some nutrients, it's packed with quickly digesting carbs that cause a blood sugar spike. For example, a 12 oz/355 ml glass of apple juice contains 48 grams of carbs- more than soda, which contains 39 g. Additionally, a 12 oz/355 ml serving of grape juice contains 60 grams of carbs.

Finally, juice is liquid carbs, so your brain doesn't process it in the same way that it does solid carbs. When you drink juices, it can actually cause you to be hungrier and end up eating more later on during the day.

Low-Fat/Fat-Free Salad Dressings

Since salads are made up of non-starchy veggies, you can enjoy a plethora of salads when you're on a low carb diet. However, you should be aware that the low-fat/fat free salad dressings actually add more carbs than you might think. For example:

- 2 Tbsp/30 ml Fat-Free French Dressing: 10 grams carbs
- 2 Tbsp/30 ml Fat-Free Ranch Dressing: 11 grams carbs

The worst part is that even though the suggested serving size is 2 Tbsp/30 ml, most people actually use more than that- especially on a large salad. If you want to decrease your carb count, it's best to use a creamy, full-fat dressing instead. On the other hand, you might want to consider simply using olive oil and vinegar- which, according to experts, has been proven to improve the health of your heart and could potentially assist in weight loss.

Beans/Legumes

Beans/legumes are high in nutrition and have many benefits, including decreasing inflammation and your risk for heart disease- but they are high in carbs. Depending upon your carb limits, these could be included in your low carb diet.

Following are the carb counts for one serving of cooked beans/legumes:

- Lentils: 40 grams carbs/16 g from fiber
- Peas: 25 grams carbs/9 g from fiber
- Black beans: 41 grams carbs/15 g from fiber
- Pinto beans: 45 grams carbs/15 g from fiber
- Chickpeas: 45 grams carbs/12 g from fiber
- Kidney beans: 40 grams carbs/13 g from fiber

As you can see, beans/legumes are healthy- but are high in carbs. However, you don't have to necessarily cut them out completely, you can consume small amounts, depending upon your personal carb limits.

Honey/Sugar (any kind)

You already know that foods containing white sugar, such as cakes, candy, and cookies are a "no-go" on a low carb diet. What you may not be aware of is that even natural forms of sugar can have as many- if not more- carbs than white sugar when you measure them in tablespoons. Following are the carbohydrate counts for 1 Tbsp of various types of sugar:

- White sugar: 12.6 g
- Maple syrup: 13 g
- Agave nectar: 16 g
- Honey: 17 g

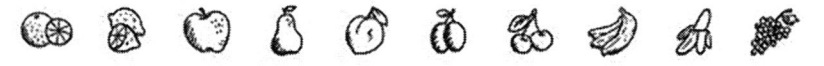

Additionally, these don't really bring any other nutritional value to the table. When you are limiting your carbs, it's critical that you choose sources that are nutritious and high in fiber. In order to sweeten foods/drinks without increasing carb count, choose a healthy sweetener.

Chips/Crackers

When it comes to snack time, many people reach for chips and/or crackers. However, the carbs from these foods can add up quite quickly. An average serving size of tortilla chips is 10-15 chips/1 oz/28 grams and contains 18 grams carbs/1 gram from fiber. The carb counts in crackers varies depending on the way they are processed. Still, even whole wheat crackers have about 19 grams of carbs- 3 from fiber- in a 1 oz/28 gram serving. Most people consume large amounts of these snack foods in a short amount of time- so if you're on a low carb diet, it's best if you just completely avoid them.

Milk

You know that milk "does a body good"- after all, it supplies your body with various nutrients, including: B vitamins, calcium, and potassium. However, the issue is the carb count-an 8 oz/240 ml serving contains 12-13 g carbs, whether it's whole milk, low-fat, or fat-free.

Of course, if you're only using 1-2 Tbsp/15-30 ml in your coffee one time a day, you can include milk in your low-carb diet- but cream/half-and-half are much better if you drink a lot of coffee since the carb count in these are much lower. If you like to drink milk or make lattes/smoothies, you might want to substitute almond or coconut milk.

Gluten-Free Baked Goods

In recent years, gluten-free diets have become quite popular- and are necessary for those who have celiac disease, a condition that causes the gut to be inflamed when gluten is consumed. Gluten is a protein that is found in products containing rye, barley, and wheat.

So, while gluten-free is a necessary option if you have this condition, it's not the best option if you're dieting- especially if you're on a low carb diet. This is because gluten-free products typically contain more carbs than the regular versions. In addition, the flour that is used in these products often contains grains/starches that result in a glucose spike.

Therefore, if you're on a low-carb diet, you really should choose whole foods. However, if you need baked goods, bake them at home with coconut or almond flour instead of reaching for those gluten-free products.

The bottom line is this: if you're on a low-carb diet, it's necessary to choose nutritious foods that are low in carbs. As you see, some foods must be eliminated, while you can enjoy many others- as long as you practice moderation. The choices that you make depend upon your personal carb limit.

What am I Allowed to Eat?

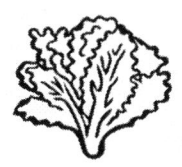

After reading the section above, you may feel like switching to a low-carb lifestyle may not be for you because there are so many things you must avoid. However, don't feel like this! There are plenty of things that you can still enjoy. In this section, you will find a list of the foods that you can still enjoy on a low-carb diet.

Meat

You can eat any type of meat that you like on a low-carb diet: beef, poultry, pork, game, and lamb. Of course, you will want to remove the skin on the chicken and you might be better to choose meats that are organic or grass fed.

Fish/Seafood

You can eat any type of seafood on a low-carb diet as well: herring, sardines, salmon, and mackerel are all great option. Additionally, since they're high in omega-3 fatty acids, they may offer some other health benefits as well. However, you will want to avoid breading them, as that will add carbs.

Eggs

If possible, you'll want to try to get organic eggs- but you can enjoy eggs cooked in any way: omelets, fried, boiled, and scrambled.

Natural Fats/High-Fat Sauces

You already know that using butter or cream when you cook makes food taste better, right? Plus, cooking this way can make you feel more satiated. Consider adding a Hollandaise or Bearnaise sauce to your meals. If you're using one that is pre-made, make sure to read the label and check for veggie oils and starches. If possible, you'll want to make it for yourself. Other good options include olive oil and coconut oil, as they are healthy fats.

Veggies

The following veggies have low carb counts, so you can enjoy them on an

y of the low-carb diet/lifestyles: asparagus, avocado, bok choy, broccoli, Brussels sprouts, cabbage, cauliflower, collards, cucumber, eggplant, kale, lettuce, mushrooms, olives, onion, peppers, spinach, tomatoes, zucchini, and other leafy greens. Of course, if you're following the keto diet, you must consume no more than 20 g carbs/day, you may want to pay attention to your portions of certain types of veggies such as Brussels sprouts and bell peppers.

Dairy

You'll want to be careful with whole, skim, and low fat milk because they contain high amounts of milk sugar. However, you can enjoy full fat options of sour cream, real butter, Greek/Turkish yogurt, cheese, and cream. All of these will keep you full and satisfied. The biggest thing to remember with dairy is to avoid low-fat, sugary, and flavored products.

Nuts

If you're craving a snack, reach for nuts instead of candy, chips, or popcorn

Berries

These are a great option, in moderation, if you are craving something sweet and you don't need to watch your carbs too closely. They're really great with whipped cream.

Drinks

It's important to stay hydrated at all times, whether you're on a low carb diet or not. However, it becomes a bit more challenging when you are on a low carb diet.

- Water is always the best choice in all situations. You can reach for sparkling or flavored water if you wish, but you'll want to double check the labels for added sugars, as well as the carb count.
- Coffee/Tea is an acceptable option but needs to be plain or with a small amount of milk/cream. If you drink coffee throughout the day, you'll want to avoid adding a lot of milk/cream when you're not hungry. You can use butter and coconut oil or full-fat cream when you're hungry.

Celebrations/Special Events

What if you're celebrating or you've been invited out with friends? Don't worry too much about it, you don't have to completely go off the rails with your diet. Sure, it's true that a lot of celebrating can slow your progress if you're trying to lose weight, just get back to your diet as soon as you can and you'll continue to lose weight.

- Alcohol: you can enjoy alcohol such as sparkling wine, champagne, gin, dry wine, whisky, vodka, and brandy in moderation.
- Chocolate: chocolate is not off limits on a low carb diet, but needs to be dark chocolate, more than 70% cocoa, and only in small amounts.
- Dark chocolate: small amounts of 70% or higher cocoa

How Many Carbs Should I Consume Each Day?

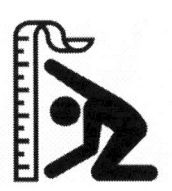

Before we start to explore the low-carb lifestyle, you'll want to take the time to determine your personal daily carb limit so that you can know how much you can comfortably cut back to. When you ask how many carbs you should be consuming, you'll probably get an answer like this: It depends. While this isn't really an exciting answer, it's the best one because after all, the carbs that you need is determined by your body's makeup, your activity level, and whether or not you have any underlying medical issues. In addition, your needs may fluctuate, depending on were you are in your cycle or the time of year.

Individuals with SAD, or seasonal affective disorder, are likely to reach for carb-rich foods during the darker months, due to the fact that their serotonin dips. Carb consumption helps with serotonin production, which explains why we crave carbs on emotionally draining days.

According to the 2015-2020 Dietary Guidelines, 45-65% of our daily calories should be from carbs. This means that on the typical 2,000 calorie diet, we should be consuming 225-325 grams. The minimum recommended amount of carbs is 130 grams, which is about eight to nine 15-gram servings daily.

If you're interested in starting a low-carb diet and you want to track your macronutrients, you can make changes to your carb:protein:fat ratio until you find the balance that allows you to meet your goals but also feels sustainable. Keep in mind that if you're not consuming enough carbs, you will typically feel mentally drained and sluggish. Additionally, you may have a hard time keeping yourself together emotionally. On the other hand, if you consume too many carbs, you don't stay full for very long because your body is burning through your meals/snacks quickly. This is the cause of the "blood sugar roller coaster", which could potentially result in insulin resistance and prediabetes.

It's best to include carbs in every meal. The way that you incorporate them is entirely up to you. However, when you spread your carbs out through the day, you keep your glucose levels stable, which balances your mood and energy levels.

How to Get Started on a Low Carb Eating Plan

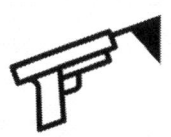

So far, we have explored what carbs are, how they react in our body, and what low carb really means. In this section, we will take a look at the steps you'll need to follow in order to get started on a low carb diet/lifestyle.

As you can see, low carb diets are conducive to weight loss. However, when it comes right down to it, it's a bit daunting to do. If you are like most, it is going to require some drastic changes and significant commitment. While there's tons of information out there, you need some practical tips that you can easily incorporate into your life.

First of all, you must start by slowly reducing your consumption of simple carbs and increasing your consumption of complex carbs. Once you've done that, you can start making some low-carb swaps. Additionally, keep in mind that you can make smarter meal choices to keep you fuller longer. If you plan on sticking with this low carb eating plan for the long haul, you'll want to do some research and settle on a specific diet plan so that you can have access to helpful tools and a community of others for support.

Reduce Carb Consumption

When it comes to reducing your carb consumption, the very first thing you must do is cut out all simple carbohydrates and refined sugars. Of course, you should not cut them out all at once, that would be too much. In order to make the process more bearable, it's best to cut them out one at a time. Start by replacing sugary drinks/sodas with sugar-free drinks and water. Some popular sources of simple carbs/refined sugars include: candy, white bread, sodas/sugary drinks, cookies/cakes/baked goods, white rice, pasta, and potatoes.

As you transition away from these simple carbohydrates and refined sugars, switch to whole grains. Before you go all in with the low-carb way of life, consider replacing some of your simple carbs with whole grain options. Once again, start out slowly, replacing one serving of your typical carbohydrate with a whole grain option every day for about one week. After a week or so, you'll find that you're not eating nearly as many simple carbs and choosing more complex carbs. This reduces your overall carb consumption, and (bonus!) you'll feel full and satisfied longer. Here are a few complex carb options to keep in mind: steel-cut oatmeal, brown rice, high-fiber/low-sugar cereal, and whole wheat pastas and breads.

As stated previously, white potatoes are considered a simple carb. Therefore, as you transition into your new low-carb lifestyle, you'll want to swap them for sweet potatoes/root veggies. You can bake/use sweet potatoes and other root veggies just as you would white potatoes. Some great options include the following: baked sweet potatoes/yams, mashed turnips/rutabaga, roasted beets/carrots/kohlrabi, and celery root/daikon radish fries.

When you're ready to transition into your new low carb lifestyle/diet, it's best to try simple swaps to decrease your carb consumption. Here are a few simple swaps you can make that won't leave you feeling deprived of your favorite foods:

- Instead of white rice, choose cauliflower rice. Take your food processor/box grater and shred a head of cauliflower into rice-like chunks. You can then cook it by microwaving for 3 to 4 minutes and then use it for any recipe that calls for rice.
- Instead of pasta noodles, use spaghetti squash or zucchini noodles. You can use a vegetable peeler/mandoline slicer to make zucchini noodles or bake spaghetti squash, scoop out seeds and scape out strands. Then, top with your favorite pasta sauce and enjoy.

- Instead of snacking on potato chips, munch on raw veggies or nuts instead. There are times when you need something crunchy to snack on- but instead of wasting those calories on potato chips, choose something healthy, such as a handful of nuts or fresh carrots or celery.
- Instead of reaching for candy or baked goods, choose berries. They are low in carbs, but high in other nutrients. Plus, they're as sweet- if not sweeter- than candy. If you have a craving for something sweet, grab a handful of raspberries, strawberries, or blueberries.

Stay Full & Satisfied

When you switch to a new way of eating, it can be difficult to stay full and satisfied. After all, you're used to eating those simple carbs- all day long. However, when you cut back on carbs, you have to make more of an effort to make good food choices. Even though you won't be eating as much, these tips will ensure you stay full and satisfied.

Proteins should be the primary focus of your meals- but that can lead to cholesterol issues, right? Choose lean proteins that have lower fat content such as the following: canned tuna in water, tofu, ground turkey, egg whites, skinless chicken, cottage cheese (low-fat), or lean ground beef.

While you do have to cut back on starchy veggies on low-carb diets, most of them will allow you to eat an unlimited amount of non-starchy veggies, which help keep you full. Here are a few options to choose from: broccoli, cabbage, cauliflower, cucumbers, eggplant, peppers, spinach, and zucchini.

For many people, snacking is a major problem when switching to a low carb diet- but you can keep yourself full and satisfied by stocking your fridge/pantry with plenty of low carb snack options. Here are a few great options: beef jerky, plain Greek yogurt, fresh veggies (such as broccoli, celery, peppers, etc), boiled eggs, or raw almonds.

Making the effort to stay hydrated on a low carb diet will also do wonders for helping you feel full and satisfied- plus, it will help you avoid dehydration. The best option is to drink water and unsweetened drinks because when you drink sugar-free sodas/ artificially sweetened drinks, it can actually trigger your sweet tooth, which is not something you want. Here are a few great beverage options: coffee, unsweetened tea, or sparkling water.

Choose a Diet You Can Stick With Long-Term

Since the low carb movement has gained so much popularity, there are several options to choose from when it comes to diets. However, you want to do some research and find one that works for you for the long term. You don't want to bounce around from diet to diet- you want something that you can make work for you. Here is a little bit of information on some of the more popular ones:

Atkins

If you want a classic low-carb diet, Atkins is an excellent choice. It has been around for a few years and many people have been successful on it, which means it's a great place to start your low-carb journey. According to Atkins experts, you can lose around 15 pounds (6.8 kg) within the first two weeks you're on it. Therefore, if you need to quickly shed a lot of weight, this is a great plan.

Getting Started with Atkins

For the first two weeks, you will have to cut down to 20 g carbs/day. In addition, you'll have to completely eliminate refined sugars/simple carbs. Other things you'll have to cut out the first two weeks are: starchy veggies such as corn, potatoes, and broccoli; nuts and whole grains. As you continue following the Atkins plan, you'll add these in slowly.

Atkins requires that you have some form of protein with every meal. You can keep things interesting by trying something new every few nights. Take some time to experiment with turkey, fish, chicken, and even tofu.

Atkins is great for those who struggle with health conditions such as high blood pressure, cardiovascular disease, metabolic syndrome, or diabetes. There are some claims that Atkins has improved these conditions- and some have even claimed that Atkins reversed their condition.

South Beach Diet

If your primary goal for going low carb is to develop healthy eating habits, you might want to consider the South Beach Diet. A cardiologist developed the South Beach Diet and it will not only help with weight loss, but also encourages healthy eating habits. Another good thing about the South Beach Diet is that it doesn't restrict carbs as much as some of the other diet plans, so many people find that it's much easier to stick to in the long run.

Getting Started with South Beach Diet
1. **Phase 1:** Cut out all carbs
2. **Phase 2:** Begin to slowly re-introduce healthy carbs into your diet (1-2 servings/day)
3. **Phase 3:** Add carbs back into your diet- practicing the art of moderation

The South Beach Diet does guide you to choose carbs with a low glycemic index, which will help moderate your hunger and blood sugar. Also, this diet encourages you to choose monosaturated fats, which are heart-healthy. Finally, the South Beach Diet promotes fruit (in moderation), veggies, and lean proteins.

Ketogenic Diet

Lately, the ketogenic diet is extremely popular, and is great for those who want a meal plan that is both satisfying and high in fat. The focus of this plan is to increase your daily calories to the following: 75% fat, 5% carbs, and 20% protein, which encourages your body to use up your fat stores, leading to quick weight loss.

According to the experts, the ketogenic diet has been proven to benefit those who have been diagnosed with epilepsy- but it may also help with the prevention of dementia, Alzheimer's, and stroke and help people heal from traumatic brain injury. However, there are potential side effects such as moodiness, brain fog, and fatigue as you change your eating habits.

Dukan Diet

If you need a structured plan to get you started in your new low-carb lifestyle, try the Dukan diet. It's one of the most structured plans you'll find. For the first ten days of this diet plan, you're only allowed to eat oat bran, lean protein, and drink water. After ten days, you can add non-starchy veggies, hard cheese, one serving of fruit, and a serving of whole grains. According to the experts, you may lose 10 pounds/4.5 kg in the first two weeks, and about 2 to 4 pounds/0.91 to 1.8 kg after that.

Of course, one of the issues with the Dukan diet is the restrictions. You are at risk for some nutritional deficiencies.

Paleo Diet

Another popular option is the Paleo diet, which is a great option if you want to put emphasis on whole foods. On this diet, you must cut out all processed foods, dairy, potatoes, and grains. You can eat your fill of fruits, roots, veggies, nuts, and meat- which will help you stay full and satisfied. This plan is healthy because of the emphasis on whole foods.

Paleo diet experts believe that many of today's health issues are due to our diet, which include lots of grains and dairy.

Stay Healthy & Motivated

The hardest part of any lifestyle change is staying motivated. However, it can be done- just keep the following in mind:

If you have a diagnosed medical condition, be sure to speak with your physician before making any changes to your diet. They will be able to advise you on whether a low carb diet is good for your situation. Additionally, they can help you choose the right one.

For example, if you have been diagnosed with diabetes, it's probably best if you swap out healthy carbs such as whole grains and fruits, instead of eliminating all carbs. If you have high cholesterol, it's not good to choose foods high in saturated fats and cholesterol. Your physician suggest that you choose lean proteins: egg whites, skinless poultry, and low-fat cottage cheese.

One great way to keep up with your carbs, is to use a tracking app. Of course, you will have to be committed to logging everything you eat. This will help you keep track of the carbs/macros you're consuming. Some apps even have a function where you can store recipes, make grocery lists, and even plan meals.

On the other hand, some people prefer to write things down- and there's nothing wrong with that. Simply grab a journal/notebook and write down everything each day. You can use the food labels to find the nutrition information. If there's not a food label, take the time to look up the calories, carbs, protein, and fat in a guidebook or online.

One way to keep yourself on track is to take the time to prep meals ahead of time. Simply set aside a few hours one day to find a few recipes and put together some (if not all) of your meals for the week. This way, you're less likely to come home after a long day at work and choose unhealthy take out over a healthier at home option. Here are a few tips for prepping your meals ahead of time:

- Prep ingredients. Take time to chop up any veggies that you need for your meals during the week. Then, measure them out and place them in separate containers for cooking.

- Cook proteins. If possible, go ahead and cook your proteins so that you just need to heat them up when you're ready. Bake salmon, grill chicken, boil eggs, and prepare other protein as desired.

- Portion meals. Take the time to portion your meals into single serving containers so that you can grab and go. An example would be 4 oz/35 g grilled chicken (skinless), 1 c/91 g steamed broccoli, and 1 c/150 g baked zucchini.

Many people find their motivation to keep going by connecting with a community of others who are following the same diet. This will give you somewhere to turn when you have questions or concerns about starting or sticking to the diet. They can give you tips/advice- and you can help them as well. You can find communities online or in your local area. However, when you join, don't just sit idle- get involved!

When you join, introduce yourself and let them know that you're just getting started and you could use some help. When you struggle, don't hesitate to reach out to others for some support. For example, if you're struggling with sweet cravings, ask others what they've done to combat those cravings. Chances are, they've been there (or maybe still are) and can offer you some advice.

LOW CARB RECIPES

Low Carb Breakfast Recipes

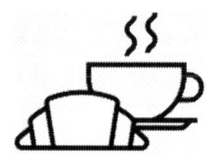

GOAT CHEESE & HERB OMELET

Time: 10 mins | Serves 1
Nutrition Information:
Calories: 523/Calories from fat: 387 | Fat: 24 g | Cholesterol: 709 mg
Protein: 31 g | Carbs: 3 g

What You Need:

- 3 eggs
- 1 Tbsp butter, unsalted
- 2 oz fresh goat cheese
- 1 Tbsp chopped herbs such as basil, cilantro, or parsley
- Salt & black pepper (to taste)

What to Do:

9. In a bowl, whisk together eggs, salt, pepper, and herbs.
10. In skillet, melt butter.
11. Once hot, add eggs and cook about 3-4 mins- until set.
12. Crumble goat cheese and fold over.
13. Cook until cheese is melty- about 1 min.

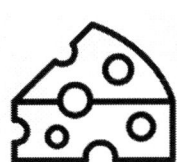

FRITTATA WITH SPINACH & GOAT CHEESE

> *Nutrition Information:*
> *Calories: 399 | Fat: 31 g | Cholesterol: 551 mg*
> *Protein: 23 g | Carbohydrates: 9 g*

What You'll Need:

- 3 Tbsps olive oil
- ½ medium-size onion, sliced thin
- 5 oz (6 cups) baby spinach
- 10 large eggs
- 4 oz (1 cup) goat cheese crumbles
- 1 Tbsp white wine vinegar
- 5 oz (6 cups) mixed greens
- Kosher salt/black pepper (to taste)
- Country bread

What You'll Do:

1. Preheat oven to 400°F/204°C.
2. In medium nonstick, ovenproof skillet, heat 1 Tbsp olive oil.
3. Place onion, along with salt & pepper in skillet and saute until golden- about 3-4 mins.
4. Add baby spinach and cook until wilted, 1-2 mins.
5. Add eggs and sprinkle goat cheese on top. Cook until eggs begin to set around edges, 1-2 mins.
6. Place in oven and bake until set, about 10-12 mins.
7. In a large bowl, whisk together remaining 2 Tbsp oil, salt & pepper, and vinegar.
8. Add mixed greens, tossing to combine. Serve with country bread and frittata.

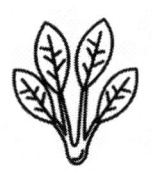

FRIED EGG SANDWICH

Total Time: 21 mins | Servings: 1
Nutrition Information:
Calories: 477 | Fat: 36 g | Carbs: 1 g
*Protein: 34 g | **Cholesterol: 450 mg***
What You'll Need:

- Nonstick cooking spray
- 3 slices bacon
- Salt & black pepper, to taste
- 2 eggs
- 1/3 c shredded cheddar cheese

What You'll Do:

1. In skillet, brown bacon on medium high heat- about 10 mins.
2. Drain grease onto paper towels. Crumble, set aside.
3. In separate skillet, cook eggs until whites are set and firm- approximately 3-4 mins.
4. Flip and continue cooking.
5. Sprinkle bacon & cheese over one egg.
6. Continue cooking until eggs reach desired doneness and cheese is melty.
7. Place second egg on top and move to serving dish.

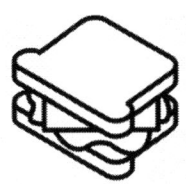

SPINACH QUICHE (NO CRUST)

Total Time: 50 mins | Servings: 6
Nutrition Information:
Calories: 309 | Fat: 23 g | Carbs: 4 g
Protein: 20 g | Cholesterol: 209 mg

What You'll Need:

- 1 Tbsp vegetable oil
- 5 eggs
- 1 onion, chopped
- Salt & black pepper, as desired
- 3 c shredded muenster cheese
- 10-oz bag frozen (thawed/drained) spinach, chopped

What You'll Do:

1. Preheat oven to 350°F/175°C.
2. Lightly grease 9-inch pie pan.
3. Place oil in skillet and heat on med-high heat. Add onions, cook until soft.
4. Add spinach and cook until excess moisture is evaporated.
5. In separate bowl, combine salt, pepper, eggs, and cheese.
6. Stir in spinach and place mixture in pie pan.
7. Place in oven and bake about 30 mins, or until eggs have set.
8. Cool for 10 mins before serving.

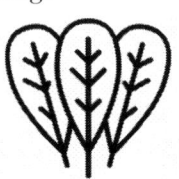

EGG & CHEESE BOATS

Total Time: 43 mins | Servings: 2
Nutrition Information:
Calories: 578 | Fat: 44 g | Carbs: 7 g
Protein: 38 g | Cholesterol: 482 mg

What You'll Need:

- 4 eggs
- 2 oval sandwich rolls
- 3 Tbsp whole milk
- 1 (4-oz) can chopped green chili peppers
- 1 c shredded cheddar cheese
- ½ c pepper Jack cheese, shredded
- ½ tsp smoked paprika
- ¼ tsp salt

What You'll Do:

1. Preheat oven to 350°F/175°C.
2. Use parchment paper to line baking sheet.
3. Cut a v-shape in each roll, but leave the ends together.
4. Lift out the wedge and hollow out rolls to make bread bowls.
5. Take care that you don't cut through the bottom or sides of the rolls.
6. Place rolls on baking sheet.
7. Crack eggs and pour milk into separate bowl and whisk until blended.
8. Stir in chili peppers, cheeses, salt, and paprika.
9. Slowly pour into prepared rolls, using a spoon to spread evenly.
10. Bake for 20 mins or until set and cheese is browned.
11. Allow to cool for 3 mins before serving.

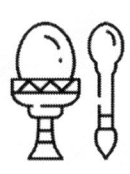

SAUSAGE CASSEROLE

> Total Time: 1 h 45 mins | Servings: 12
> Nutrition Information:
> Calories: 355 | Fat: 26 g | Carbs: 8 g
> Protein: 21 g | Cholesterol: 188 mg

What You'll Need:

- 1 lb breakfast sausage, sage flavored
- 3 c shredded potatoes,
- ¼ c melted butter
- 12 oz shredded cheddar cheese
- ½ c shredded onion
- 1 (16-oz) container cottage cheese, small curd
- 6 jumbo eggs

What You'll Do:

1. Preheat oven to 375°F/190°C.
2. Grease 9x13 baking dish.
3. Brown sausage in skillet over med-high heat until evenly browned. Drain. Set aside.
4. In baking dish, stir butter and potatoes together. Line sides and bottom with potatoes.
5. Mix onion, eggs, sausage, cheese, and cottage cheese in separate bowl and pour over potatoes.
6. Bake for about 1 hour.
7. Allow to rest for 5 mins before cutting and serving.

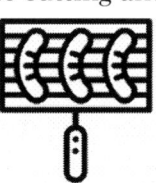

OVEN SCRAMBLED EGGS

Total Time: 35 mins | Servings: 12
Nutrition Information:
Calories: 236 | Fat: 18 g | Carbs: 3 g
Protein: 14 g | Cholesterol: 396 mg

What You'll Need:

- ½ c melted butter/margarine
- 24 eggs
- ¼ tsp salt
- ½ c milk

What You'll Do:

1. Preheat oven to 350°F/175°C.
2. Pour melted butter into baking dish.
3. In separate bowl, whisk eggs and salt until blended. Slowly blend in milk.
4. Pour into baking dish and place in oven, uncovered for 10 mins.
5. After 10 mins, stir and bake for 10-15 additional mins, or until eggs are set.

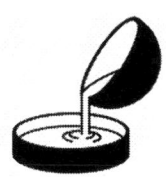

OVEN-BAKED DENVER OMELET

> *Total Time: 45 mins | Servings: 4*
> *Nutrition Information:*
> *Calories: 345 | Fat: 26 g | Carbs: 3 g*
> *Protein: 22 g | Cholesterol: 381 mg*

What You'll Need:
- 2 Tbsp butter
- ½ each green bell pepper & onion, chopped
- 1 c chopped cooked ham
- 8 eggs
- ¼ c milk
- ½ c cheddar cheese, shredded
- Salt & black pepper, to taste

What You'll Do:
1. Preheat oven to 400°F/200°C.
2. Grease 10-in round baking dish.
3. Over medium heat, melt butter in skillet.
4. Cook bell pepper and onion about 5 mins.
5. Add ham and continue to cook until heated through, about 5 more mins.
6. In separate bowl, combine milk and eggs.
7. Add ham & cheese mixture and season as desired.
8. Pour into prepared baking dish.
9. Bake until eggs are puffy & brown, about 25 mins. Serve warm.

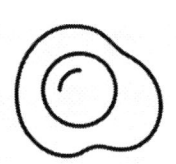

HAM, CHEESE, & HASHBROWN CASSEROLE

> *Total Time: 1 hr 15 mins | Servings: 12*
> *Nutrition Information:*
> *Calories: 415 | Fat: 27 g | Carbs: 30 g*
> *Protein: 14 g | Cholesterol: 53 mg*

What You'll Need:

- 1 (32-oz) package frozen hash browns
- 8 ounce cooked ham, diced
- 2 c shredded sharp cheddar cheese
- 1 ½ c grated paremesan
- 2 (10.75 oz) cans cream of potato soup
- 16-oz sour cream

Directions

1. Preheat oven to 375°F/190°C.
2. Lightly grease 9x13 casserole dish.
3. In separate bowl, mix cheddar cheese, soup, hash browns, sour cream, and ham.
4. Spread mixture into casserole dish and sprinkle parmesan on top.
5. Bake until bubbly and light brown- about 1 hour.

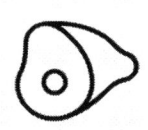

FRENCH TOAST

Total Time: 30 mins | Servings: 12
Nutrition Information:
Calories: 123 | Fat: 2 g | Carbs: 18
Protein: 5 g | Cholesterol: 48 mg

What You'll Need:

- ¼ c flour, all purpose
- 1 c milk
- 1 pinch salt
- 3 eggs
- ½ tsp cinnamon
- 1 tsp vanilla extract
- 1 Tbsp white sugar
- 12 slices bread

What You'll Do:

1. Put flour into large mixing bowl and slowly add milk.
2. Then add eggs, salt, vanilla extract, cinnamon, and sugar until mixture is smooth.
3. Place pan/griddle on medium heat.
4. Soak bread in mixture until saturated.
5. Cook until golden brown.

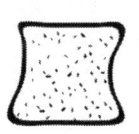

Low Carb Lunch Recipes

CHIPPED BEEF ON TOAST

Total Time: 20 mins | Servings: 4
Nutrition Information:
Calories: 197 | Fat: 9 g | Carbs: 9 g
Protein: 21 g | Cholesterol: 67 mg

What You'll Need:

- 2 Tbsp butter
- 2 Tbsp flour, all-purpose
- ½ c milk, warm
- 1 (8-oz) jar dried beef
- 1 pinch cayenne pepper

What You'll Do:

1. On low heat, melt butter in medium-size saucepan.
2. Whisk in flour to create roux.
3. Slowly add milk and increase to med-high heat. Continue to cook until mixture has thickened and bring to a boil.
4. Then, stir in cayenne and beef and heat through. Serve on toast.

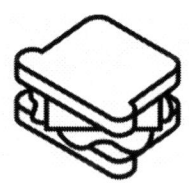

LOW CARB BURGER

> Total Time: 20 mins | Servings: 6
> Nutrition Information:
> Calories: 323 | Fat: 17 g | Carbs: 10 g
> Protein: 30 g | Cholesterol: 122 mg

What You'll Need:

- 2 lbs ground beef, extra lean
- 1 (1 Oz) package onion soup mix
- 1 egg
- 2 tsp each Worcestershire sauce and hot sauce
- ¼ tsp black pepper
- ¾ c rolled oats

What You'll Do:

1. Preheat outdoor grill and lightly oil grate.
2. In small bowl, lightly beat egg.
3. In a separate large bowl, combine beef, egg, oats, onion soup mix, and hot sauce.
4. Create 6 patties from mixture.
5. Place patties on grill and grill on med-high heat for 10-20 mins, until they reach desired doneness.

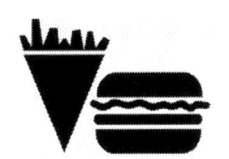

BEEF DIP SANDWICH

> Total Time: 6 h 10 mins | Servings: 10
> Nutrition Information:
> Calories: 290 | Fat: 20 g | Carbs: 2 g (more if eaten on bread)
> Protein: 23 g | Cholesterol: 82 mg

What You'll Need:

- 4 lbs beef chuck roast
- 1 Tbsp garlic, minced
- 1 Tbsp dried rosemary
- 3 bay leaves
- 1 c soy sauce
- 6 c water

What You'll Do:

1. Season roast with garlic and rosemary.
2. Place roast and bay leaves in slow cooker and pour water and soy sauce in.
3. Cook on low for 6-10 hours.
4. Keep in mind, with this roast, the longer it cooks, the better it is.
5. When roast is done, remove from slow cooker and shred. Enjoy with or without bread.

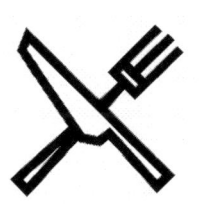

GARLIC SALMON

> Total Time: 40 mins | Servings: 6
> Nutrition Information:
> Calories: 169 | Fat: 7 g | Carbs: 2 g
> Protein: 24 g | Cholesterol: 50 mg

What You'll Need:

- 1 ½ lbs salmon filet
- Salt & black pepper (to taste)
- 3 cloves garlic, minced
- 1 sprig fresh dill
- 5 sprigs fresh dill weed
- 5 slices lemon
- 2 green onions, chopped

What You'll Do:

1. Preheat oven to 450°F/230°C and spray 2 large pieces of foil with cooking spray.
2. Place salmon on top of one piece of foil.
3. Sprinkle with garlic, chopped dill, salt, and pepper.
4. Arrange lemon on top and place one sprig of dill weed on top of each lemon.
5. Sprinkle with chopped green onion.
6. Cover with second piece of foil and pinch together to seal.
7. Place in large baking dish.
8. Bake for 20-25 mins, until flaky.

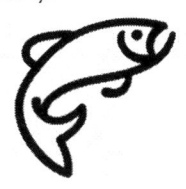

BACON & FETA STUFFED CHICKEN BREASTS

Total Time: 45 mins | Servings: 4
Nutrition Information:
Calories: 451 | Fat: 35 g | Carbs: 3 g
Protein: 32 g | Cholesterol: 93 mg

What You'll Need:

- 8 Tbsp olive oil
- 4 chicken breasts (boneless/skinless)
- 2 tsp lemon juice
- 1 Tbsp oregano
- 4 cloves garlic, crushed
- Salt & black pepper (as desired)
- 4 slices each bacon (fried/drained) and feta cheese

What You'll Do:

1. Preheat oven to 350°F/175°C.
2. In small bowl, mix together salt, pepper, lemon juice, oil, oregano, and garlic.
3. Slice chicken breasts halfway through to make an opening to place bacon and feta into.
4. Line 9x13 inch baking dish with foil and place chicken in dish.
5. Stuff each one with 1 slice each bacon and feta.
6. Secure open sides with toothpicks.
7. Drizzle with lemon juice mixture and place in oven.
8. Bake uncovered for about 30 mins.

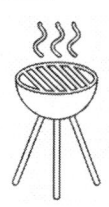

TURKEY BURGERS WITH FETA CHEESE

> Total Time: 20 mins | Servings: 4
> Nutrition Information:
> Calories: 318 | Fat: 22 g | Carbs: 4 g
> Protein: 26 g | Cholesterol: 123 mg

What You'll Need:

- 1 lb ground turkey
- 1 c feta cheese, crumbled
- ½ c kalamata olives, pitted & sliced
- 2 tsp oregano
- Black pepper (to taste)

What You'll Do:

1. Preheat grill to med-high and lightly oil grate.
2. In large bowl, mix together ground turkey, black pepper, oregano, feta cheese, and olives.
3. Form 4 patties from mixture.
4. Place patties on grill and cook for 10-12 mins, flipping over halfway through cook time.

HAM & CHEESE ROLLS

Total Time: 35 mins | Servings: 24
Nutrition Information:
Calories: 145 | Fat: 9 g | Carbs: 10 g
Protein: 6 g | Cholesterol: 18 mg

What You'll Need:

- 2 Tbsp minced onion
- 1 Tbsp mustard
- 2 Tbsp poppy seeds
- ½ c melted margarine
- 24 dinner rolls
- ½ lb ham, chopped
- ½ lb Swiss cheese, thinly sliced

What You'll Do:

1. Preheat oven to 325°F/165°C.
2. In small bowl, mix together margarine, mustard, onion flakes, and poppy seeds.
3. Split each dinner roll and place ham and cheese inside to make a sandwich.
4. Arrange rolls on baking sheet and dribble melted margarine on top.
5. Bake until cheese is melty- about 20 mins.

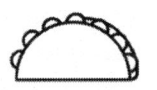

BBQ BACON SHRIMP

Total Time: 45 mins | Servings: 3
Nutrition Information:
Calories: 160 | Fat: 11 g | Carbs: 0.3 g
Protein: 15 g | Cholesterol: 83 mg

What You'll Need:

- 16 large shrimp, peeled/deveined
- 8 slices bacon
- BBQ seasoning

What You'll Do:

1. Preheat oven to 450°F/230°C.
2. Wrap shrimp with ½ slice bacon, secure with toothpick. Note: make sure to use large shrimp, as the cook time on the shrimp and bacon is similar. If you use medium-size shrimp, you'll want to precook your bacon, as overcooked shrimp are rubbery/tough.
3. Line pan with foil and place baking rack in pan.
4. Put shrimp on rack and sprinkle with BBQ seasoning.
5. Flip shrimp and sprinkle other side.
6. Let sit for about 15 mins so that seasonings can soak in.
7. Bacon will turn opaque, instead of being creamy white.
8. Bake in oven until bacon is crisp & shrimp tender, about 10-15 mins.

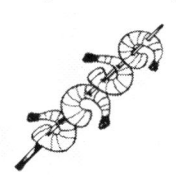

GRILLED MUSHROOMS

Total Time: 35 mins | Servings: 4
Nutrition Information:
Calories: 156 | Fat: 14 g | Carbs: 7 g
Protein: 3 g | Cholesterol: 0 mg

What You'll Need:

- ½ c red bell pepper, finely chopped
- 1 garlic clove, minced
- ¼ c olive oil
- ¼ tsp onion powder
- Salt & black pepper, as desired
- 4 portobello mushroom caps

What You'll Do:

1. Preheat grill to medium and lightly oil grate.
2. In large bowl, combine black pepper, salt, garlic, red bell pepper, onion powder, and oil.
3. Spread on grill side of mushroom caps.
4. Place mushrooms to the side (over indirect heat) and cover.
5. Cook for 15-20 mins.

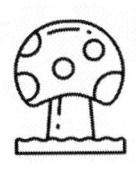

GRILLED TANDOORI CHICKEN

Total Time: 8 h 55 mins | Servings: 8
Nutrition Information:
Calories: 349 | Fat: 21 g | Carbs: 5 g
Protein: 34 g | Cholesterol: 120 mg

What You'll Need:

- 12-oz plain yogurt
- Salt and black pepper, as desired
- ½ tsp ground cloves
- 2 Tbsp ginger, fresh grated
- 3 cloves garlic, finely minced
- 4 tsp paprika
- 2 tsp each cinnamon, coriander, and cumin
- 16 chicken thighs
- Olive oil spray

What You'll Do:

1. In medium bowl, combine ginger, salt, cloves, pepper, and yogurt.
2. Add coriander, cinnamon, garlic, cumin, and paprika and set aside.
3. Under cold water, carefully rinse chicken and then pat dry with paper towels and place in large zip-top bag.
4. Pour yogurt mixture over chicken and seal, making sure to press all air out of bag.
5. Turn over several times to distribute marinated evenly.
6. Place in bowl and refrigerate for 8 hours, turning occasionally.
7. Preheat grill to medium.
8. Remove chicken from bag and wipe off excess marinade.
9. Spray chicken with olive oil spray.
10. Place chicken on grill over direct heat and cook for 2 mins.

11. Then, flip and cook 2 more mins.
12. Move chicken to indirect heat and cook for 35-40 mins, until it reaches an internal temp of 180°F.

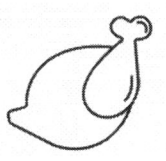

MEATBALLS W/ SWEET & SOUR SAUCE

Total Time: 1 h 50 mins | Servings: 12
Nutrition Information:
Calories: 152 | Fat: 6 g | Carbs: 17 g
Protein: 8 g | Cholesterol: 38 mg

What You'll Need:

- 12-oz can/bottle chili sauce
- 2 tsp lemon juice
- 9-oz grape jelly
- 1 lb ground beef
- 1 egg (beaten)
- 1 large onion, grated
- Salt, as desired

What You'll Do:

1. Whisk together grape jelly, lemon juice, and chili sauce.
2. Pour into slow cooker and simmer until warm.
3. Combine ground beef, salt, egg, and onion.
4. Form meatballs from mixture and add to sauce. Simmer for 1 ½ hours.

HERBY LEMON CHICKEN

> *Total Time: 25 mins | Servings: 2*
> *Nutrition Information:*
> *Calories: 212 | Fat: 9 g | Carbs: 8 g*
> *Protein: 29 g | Cholesterol: 68 mg*

What You'll Need:

- 2 chicken breast halves (boneless/skinless)
- Salt & black pepper, as desired
- 1 whole lemon
- 1 Tbsp olive oil
- 1 pinch oregano
- 2 sprigs parsley (garnish)

What You'll Do:

1. Cut lemon in half and squeeze juice from ½ onto chicken. Sprinkle with salt as desired.
2. Set aside while you heat oil in small skillet over med-low heat.
3. Once oil is heated, place chicken in skillet.
4. As you sauté, add juice from ½ lemon, oregano, and pepper to taste.
5. Sauté until juices run clear- about 5-10 mins on each side.

GYRO BURGER

Total Time: 25 mins | Servings: 4
Nutrition Information:
Calories: 338 | Fat: 25 g | Carbs: 6 g
Protein: 20 g | Cholesterol: 84 mg

What You'll Need:

- ½ lb each lean ground beef and lamb
- ½ onion, grated
- 2 cloves garlic, pressed
- 1 slice toast, crumbled
- ½ tsp each dried savory, allspice, coriander, salt, and pepper
- 1 dash cumin

What You'll Do:

1. Preheat grill to med-high and lightly oil grate.
2. In large bowl, combine bread crumbs, lamb, beef, onion, and garlic.
3. Add cumin, savory, salt, allspice, pepper, and coriander.
4. Knead until mixture is well blended and shape into 4 thin patties.
5. Cook for about 5-7 mins on each side.

Low Carb Dinner Recipes

LASAGNA STUFFED PEPPERS

Total Time: 1 h 30 mins | Servings: 12
Nutrition Facts
Calories: 232 | Fat: 13 g | Carbs: 10 g
Protein: 18 g | Cholesterol: 49 mg

What You'll Need:

- 1 lb ground beef
- 3 8-oz cans tomato sauce
- 6 bell peppers, halved & seeded
- 1 6-oz can tomato paste
- Salt (to taste)
- Water (as needed)
- 1 12-oz container cottage cheese
- Salt & black pepper, as desired
- ½ tsp oregano
- 2 c each shredded mozzarella and cheddar cheeses

What You'll Do:

1. Preheat oven to 350°F/175°C.
2. After cutting and removing the seeds from the bell peppers, place them on baking sheet- cut side up and sprinkle with salt.
3. Pour ¼ inch/0.64 cm water into pan.
4. Brown ground beef, then drain & discard grease.
5. Add 1 tsp salt, ½ tsp oregano, black pepper, tomato sauce, and tomato paste and bring to a boil.
6. Decrease heat. Simmer for about 15 mins.
7. Layer cottage cheese, mozzarella cheese, cheddar cheese, and meat sauce in each bell pepper.
8. Top with remainder of cheeses.
9. Place in oven and bake for about 50-65 mins.

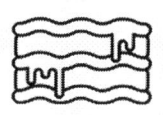

CHICKEN CACCIATORE

Total Time: 1 h 50 mins | Servings: 6
Nutrition Information:
Calories: 513 | Fat: 29 g | Carbs: 11 g
Protein: 50 g | Cholesterol: 149 mg

What You'll Need:

- Whole chicken, cut into quarters
- 2 Tbsp oil
- 1 onion
- 9 oz fresh mushrooms, quartered
- Salt & black pepper, as desired
- 4 cloves garlic, sliced
- 1 tsp oregano
- Red pepper flakes, as desired
- 3 rosemary sprigs
- 1 cup tomato sauce
- ½ c water
- 2 red/2 green bell peppers

What You'll Do:

1. Preheat oven to 350°F/175°C. On medium heat, warm olive oil in large Dutch oven.
2. Place chicken in Dutch oven and cook until outside is brown.
3. Then, place into a bowl to catch juices.
4. Add onions & mushrooms and cook until soft (about 5-6 mins).
5. Add salt, black pepper, oregano, rosemary, garlic, tomato sauce, red pepper flakes, and water.
6. Place chicken and juices back in Dutch oven on top of cooked veggies and sprinkle with more salt and black pepper.
7. Top will bell pepper slices.
8. Put lid on the Dutch oven and place in oven- cook for 1 hour 15 mins.

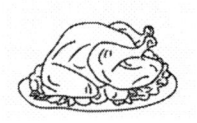

ROAST CHICKEN W/ LEMON & CARROTS

> Total Time: 1 h 25 m/Servings: 5
> Nutrition Information:
> Calories: 736 | Fat: 42 g | Carbs: 13 g
> Protein: 70 g | Cholesterol: 275 mg

What You'll Need:

- 5 lb/2.26 kg whole chicken
- Salt, to taste
- 1 onion
- 3 Tbsp olive oil
- 1 c light beer
- 1 ½ c chicken broth (more, as needed)
- 6 carrots
- 2 tsp rosemary
- 1 tsp thyme
- 1 lemon

What You'll Do:

1. Preheat oven to 425°F/220°C.
2. Using paper towels, pat chicken dry. Then, cut backbone using kitchen shears.
3. Flip chicken over, breast side up and press down to flatten. Generously season with salt.
4. Over medium heat, warm olive oil in a oven-safe cast iron skillet.
5. Place chicken skin side down and pan fry until golden, approximately 6-7 mins.
6. Transfer to plate, skin side up.
7. Add oil and onion to same skillet and cook until softened, approximately 2-3 mins. Pour beer to skillet to remove any browned bits.
8. Cook until most of the beer is reduced, approximately 2-4 mins.
9. Stir in broth, rosemary, thyme, lemon, and carrots.
10. Place chicken on top of veggies, skin side up.

11. Place in oven and roast until chicken is golden and crispy, approximately 50 mins.
12. Move chicken from pan to platter to rest.
13. Boil broth/juices about 10 mins, until thickened. Serve chicken topped with sauce.

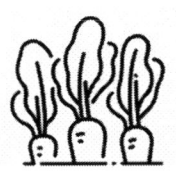

STUFFED SUMMER SQUASH

> Total Time: 55 mins | Servings: 5
> Nutrition Information:
> Calories: 148 | Fat: 10 g | Carbs: 6 g
> Protein: 8 g | Cholesterol: 24 mg

What You'll Need:

- 2 tsp olive oil
- 4 oz Merguez sausage (remove casing)
- ½ c red bell pepper, diced
- 2 oz crumbled fresh goat cheese
- 5 round summer squash, halved
- Salt & black pepper (to taste)
- 1 Tbsp dry bread crumbs (more, as needed)
- 2 tsp olive oil

What You'll Do:

1. Preheat oven to 375°F/190°C.
2. Line baking sheet with foil and coat with 1 tsp olive oil.
3. In nonstick pan over medium heat, add 1 tsp olive oil.
4. Stir in pepper and sausage and cook until sausage is brown and pepper is soft/sweet- about 7-8 mins. Drain off fat.
5. Place sausage mixture and goat cheese in bowl and mix until combined, then set aside.
6. Cut squashes in half and hollow out the centers, then place on baking sheet, cut side up.
7. Fill each with 1-2 Tbsp cheese & sausage mixture. Top with bread crumbs and drizzle with 2 tsp olive oil.
8. Bake until squash is tender and filling is golden, approximately 30 mins.

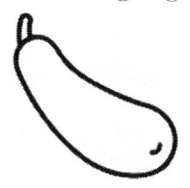

CANDIED BACON CHICKEN WITH CAULIFLOWER RICE & PECANS

Total Time: 1 h 15 min | Servings: 4
Nutrition Information:
Calories: 500 | Fat: 28 g | Carbs: 28 g
Protein: 36 g | Cholesterol: 85 mg

What You'll Need:

- 1/3 c pecans, chopped
- 2 lbs riced cauliflower
- 2 cloves garlic, grated
- 3 Tbsp oil
- 1 Tbsp thyme
- ½ tsp Kosher salt
- Black pepper, to taste
- 4 chicken breasts, sliced thin
- 8 slices bacon
- ¼ c brown sugar
- ¾ tsp chili powder
- ½ c fresh parsley, chopped

What You'll Do:

1. Toast pecans in skillet on medium heat.
2. Preheat oven to 425°F/220°C.
3. Line baking sheet with foil, making sure the foil goes up all sides to catch all juices.
4. In separate bowl, combine cauliflower, 2 tsp thyme, 1 ½ tsp salt, pepper, olive oil, and garlic, and spread on 2/3 of baking sheet. With remainder of thyme, salt, and black pepper, season chicken.
5. Wrap each chicken breast with 2 pieces of bacon, ensuring that chicken is completely covered.
6. Arrange chicken on remaining 1/3 of baking sheet.
7. Mix chili powder and brown sugar in separate bowl and sprinkle half over chicken.
8. Bake for 25 mins.

9. Stir cauliflower and flip chicken. Sprinkle remainder of brown sugar/chili powder mixture over chicken and bake until bacon is crisp and chicken is no longer pink, 20-25 mins. Your thermometer should read 165°F/74°C when inserted into chicken. If bacon needs additional crisping, turn oven to broil for a few mins.
10. Remove chicken from baking sheet and stir cauliflower into the drippings.
11. Stir in parsley and toasted pecans. Spoon into bowls and top with chicken.

LETTUCE WRAPS

> Total Time: 35 mins | Servings: 4
> Nutrition Information:
> Calories: 388 | Fat: 22 g | Carbs: 24 g
> Protein: 23 g | Cholesterol: 69 mg

What You'll Need:

- 16 lettuce leaves
- 1 Tbsp each soy sauce and oil
- 1 lb lean ground beef
- 1 onion, chopped
- ¼ c hoisin sauce
- 2 cloves garlic, minced
- 1 Tbsp rice wine vinegar
- 2 tsp pickled ginger, minced
- Asian chili pepper sauce
- 1 can (8 oz) water chestnuts
- 1 bunch finely chopped green onions
- 2 tsp sesame oil

What You'll Do:

1. Rinse lettuce leaves, pat dry, and set aside- take care that you don't tear them.
2. Place skillet on stove and heat on medium-high. Add cooking oil and beef and cook until brown & crumbly, about 5-7 mins. Drain grease and discard.
3. Place beef into separate bowl.
4. In the same skillet, cook onion until tender, about 5-10 mins. Stir in chili pepper sauce, soy sauce, garlic, vinegar, hoisin sauce, and ginger into onions.
5. Add beef, water chestnuts, sesame oil, and green onions. Cook for 2 mins.
6. To serve, pile meat mixture into the center of a serving platter and arrange lettuce leaves around.

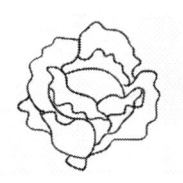

BEEF SLAW

Total Time: 31 mins | Servings: 4
Nutrition Information:
Calories: 451 | Fat: 28 g | Carbs: 26
Protein: 25 g | Cholesterol: 70 mg

What You'll Need:

- 1 Tbsp canola oil
- 4 cloves garlic, minced
- 1 Tbsp ginger, minced
- 1 lb ground beef
- 2 heads each white and red cabbage, shredded
- 2 carrots
- 1 red bell pepper
- ½ c soy sauce, reduced sodium
- 2 Tbsp sesame oil
- Dash hot sauce (or more, to taste)
- Salt & black pepper to taste
- 2 Tbsp fresh cilantro, chopped (or more, to taste)
- Lime wedge

What You'll Do:

1. Heat oil on medium heat in a large skillet/wok.
2. Add garlic & ginger, cook for 2 mins.
3. Add ground beef, cook for 6 mins.
4. Push ground beef to the side in skillet and add the red bell pepper and the shredded white and red cabbage.
5. Mix veggies with beef and cook until veggies are tender, about 5-6 mins.
6. Mix in soy sauce, hot sauce, and sesame oil until well blended.
7. Season with salt & black pepper as desired.

LASAGNA STUFFED MUSHROOMS

Total Time: 50 min | Servings: 2
Nutrition Facts
Calories: 263 | Fat: 12 g | Carbs: 9 g
Protein: 26 g | Cholesterol: 142 mg

What You'll Need:

- ¼ lb ground beef
- ½ c small curd cottage cheese, fat free
- 1 egg
- 1 Tbsp finely chopped green onion
- 1 Tbsp chopped parsley
- Salt & black pepper, to taste
- ¼ pasta sauce
- 6 large mushrooms, stems removed
- ¼ c mozzarella cheese, shredded

What You'll Do:

1. Preheat oven to 375°F/190°C.
2. Lightly coat baking pan with cooking spray.
3. Place ground beef in skillet and cook for about 10 mins.
4. In a separate bowl, mix salt & pepper, green onion, cottage cheese, parsley, and egg until well blended- add ground beef.
5. Place mushrooms in baking sheet, hollow sides up. Add approximately 1 Tbsp of the filling into each one, allowing remainder to overflow between them.
6. Bake until filling is set, approximately 15 mins.
7. Remove from oven and spread pasta sauce over the top.
8. Sprinkle mozzarella cheese on top of sauce and place back in oven.
9. Broil until cheese is beginning to brown- approximately 5 mins.

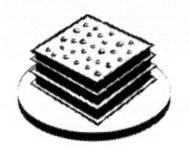

SWEET POTATO CARBONARA WITH MUSHROOMS & SPINACH

> *Total Time: 40 mins | Servings: 5*
> *Nutrition Information:*
> *Calories: 312 | Fat: 12 g | Carbs: 38 g*
> *Protein: 15 g | Cholesterol: 130 mg*

What You'll Need:

- 2 lbs sweet potatoes
- 3 jumbo eggs
- 1 c grated parmesan cheese
- 1 Tbsp olive oil
- Salt & black pepper, as desired
- 3 strips bacon, chopped
- 1 (8-oz) package mushrooms
- 2 cloves garlic, minced
- 5-oz package baby spinach

What You'll Do:

1. Bring large pot of water to a boil.
2. Using a julienne veggie peeler or spiralizer, cut sweet potatoes into long, thin strands. You should end up with around 12 cups of noodles.
3. Cook in boiling water, until beginning to soften but not totally tender- should be approximately 1 ½ to 3 mins. Drain, reserving about ¼ c of the water.
4. Place noodles back in pot, off the heat.
5. Combine reserved water, salt, black pepper, eggs, and parmesan cheese in separate bowl.
6. Pour over noodles and toss until coated evenly.
7. Over medium heat, heat oil in skillet.
8. Add bacon & mushrooms, stirring often until liquid has evaporated and mushrooms are beginning to brown.

9. Add garlic, cook for 1 min.
10. Add spinach and cook until wilted.
11. Add veggies to noodles and toss. Top with black pepper.

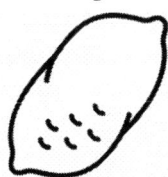

GRILLED SALMON WRAPS

> Total Time: 30 mins | Servings: 4
> Nutrition Information:
> Calories: 306 | Fat: 17 g | Carbs: 7 g
> Protein: 28 g | Cholesterol: 79 mg

What You'll Need:

Pico de Gallo:

- 1 tomato, diced and seeded
- ½ red bell pepper, diced and seeded
- ½ red onion, chopped
- Juice from 1 lime

Cream Sauce:

- 2/3 c Greek yogurt, plain
- 2 Tbsp milk, skim
- ½ tsp seasoning blend

Wraps

- 1 lb skinless salmon, grilled and cut into chunks
- 12 radicchio leaves, whole

What You'll Do:

1. To make pico de gallo, combine lime juice, red bell pepper, onion, and tomato into small bowl and set aside.
2. In a separate bowl, whisk together seasoning blend, skim milk, and Greek yogurt.
3. Place radicchio leaves on platter and place grilled chunks of salmon on top.
4. Then, top with cream sauce and pico de gallo.

PARMESAN TILAPIA

> Total Time: 15 mins | Servings: 8
> Nutrition Information:
> Calories: 224 | Fat: 12 g | Carbs: 0.8 g
> Protein: 25 g | Cholesterol: 63 mg

What You'll Need:

- ½ c parmesan cheese
- ¼ c softened butter
- 3 Tbsp mayo
- 2 Tbsp lemon juice
- ¼ tsp each dried basil and black pepper
- 1/8 tsp each celery salt and onion powder
- 2 lbs tilapia fillets

What You'll Do:

1. Preheat oven's broiler and grease broiling pan/line with foil.
2. In small bowl, combine parmesan cheese, lemon juice, mayo, and butter.
3. Season with celery salt, basil, onion powder, and black pepper.
4. Mix thoroughly and set aside.
5. Arrange tilapia fillets on prepared pan.
6. Broil a few inches from heat for 3 mins.
7. Flip fillets and broil for 2 mins.
8. Remove from oven sprinkle parmesan cheese mixture on top.
9. Put fish back in oven and broil until topping is brown/fish is flaky.

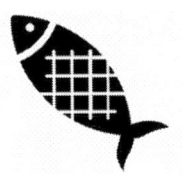

PORK CHOPS WITH MUSHROOM SAUCE

Total Time: 40 mins | Servings: 4
Nutrition Information:
Calories: 210 | Fat: 8 g | Carbs: 9 g
Protein: 23 g | Cholesterol: 65 mg

What You'll Need:

- 4 pork chops
- Salt & black pepper, as desired
- Garlic salt, as desired
- 1 onion, chopped
- ½ lb sliced mushrooms
- 1 can cream of mushroom soup

What You'll Do:

1. Season chops with garlic salt, black pepper and salt as desired.
2. Place chops in large skillet and brown over medium heat.
3. Add mushrooms and onion, and sauté for 1 min.
4. Pour soup over chops.
5. Cover and reduce temp to med-low.
6. Simmer about 20-30 mins, until chops are tender.

Low Carb Dessert Recipes

ALMOND-RASPBERRY CUPCAKES

Total Prep Time: 40 mins | Servings: 10 cupcakes
Nutrition Information:
Calories: 237 | Fat: 20 g | Carbs: 4 g
Protein: 7 g | Fiber: 4 g

What You'll Need:

- 2 large eggs
- ¼ c butter, unsalted
- 1/3 c sweetener of choice
- 1 tsp vanilla extract
- 1 oz water
- ½ tsp fresh squeezed lemon juice
- 2 Tbsp heavy cream
- 2 Tbsp almond extract
- ½ tsp each baking powder & salt
- 2 ½ c almond or coconut flour
- 3 1/3 Tbsp red raspberry preserves, sugar free

What You'll Do:

1. Preheat oven to 350°F/176°C. Place 10 liners in muffin pan and set aside.
2. In small bowl, beat egg yolks with ¼ cup of sweetener, butter, cream, water, lemon juice, and extracts until fully combined and set aside.
3. In medium sized bowl, beat egg whites until frothy. Add remaining 2 Tbsp of sweetener and beat until stiff peaks form. Fold into egg yolk mixture.
4. In a third bowl, mix almond meal, salt, and baking powder.
5. Gently fold into egg mixture before dividing equally between the lined muffin pan.
6. Finally, drop 1 teaspoon of the raspberry jam into the center of each one.
7. Bake for 20 t0 30 mins.
8. Let cool for 20 mins in pan. You can then enjoy these warm or at room temp.

9. Store in fridge for up to one week and serve at room temp. If you want to store longer, place in freezer for up to one month.

CHOCOLATE-PEANUT BUTTER WHIP

Prep Time: 5 mins | Servings: 1
Nutrition Information:
Calories: 223 | Fat: 20 g | Carbs: 5 g
Protein: 5 g | Fiber: 3 g

What You'll Need:

- 1 Tbsp cocoa powder, unsweetened
- 1 Tbsp natural peanut butter, creamy
- 2 tsp sweetener of choice
- 2 Tbsp heavy cream

What You'll Do:

1. Blend together cocoa powder, peanut butter, and sweetener.
2. Whip heavy cream, forming soft peaks.
3. Fold whip cream into chocolate peanut butter mix.
4. If desired, use almond butter instead of peanut butter.

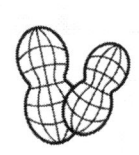

PUMPKIN PECAN CHEESECAKE

Prep Time: 1 hr 15 mins | Servings: 8
Nutrition Information:
Calories: 488 | Fat: 47 g | Carbs: 7 g
Protein: 10 g | Fiber: 3 g

What You'll Need:

Crust:

- 1 ½ c pecan halves
- 1 Tbsp sweetener
- ½ tsp cinnamon
- 2 Tbsp butter, unsalted
- 1 large egg white

Filling:

- 2 blocks (12-0z each) of cream cheese
- 2/3 c sweetener
- 1 c heavy cream
- 15 oz canned pumpkin, no salt
- 1 tsp each pumpkin pie spice and vanilla extract
- 3 large eggs, whole

What You'll Do:

Crust:

1. Preheat oven to 350°F/176°C.
2. In blender/food processor, combine pecans, 1 Tbsp sweetener, and cinnamon and process until finely ground and mixed well.
3. Add melted butter and egg white and blend just enough to combine.
4. Press mixture into 9" springform pan and bake until golden- about 8-10 mins.
5. Allow to cool on wire rack.

Filling:

1. Decrease oven temp to 325°F/162°C.
2. In a large bowl, combine cream, cream cheese, and 2/3 c sweetener, using electric mixer to blend until smooth.
3. Add canned pumpkin, pumpkin pie spice, and vanilla, mixing well.
4. Beat eggs in one at a time, until just combined.
5. Pour batter into crust and bake until just set- about 45-50 mins.
6. Turn oven off and allow pie to stand for 10 mins.
7. Move to wire rack and cool completely. Cover and put in fridge until chilled. Slice and serve.

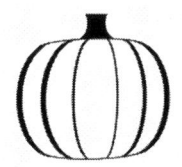

VANILLA ALMOND BUTTER COOKIES

> Nutrition Information:
> Calories: 55 | Fat: 4 g
> Protein: 2 g | Carbs: 2 g | Fiber: 0.7 g

What You'll Need:

- 1 ½ c almonds, slivered and blanched
- ¾ c soy flour, whole grain
- 3 Tbsp baking powder
- ¾ c sweetener
- 1 large whole egg & 1 large egg yolk
- 2 Tbsp vanilla extract
- ¼ c butter, unsalted

What You'll Do:

1. Preheat oven to 375°F/190°C.
2. In blender/food processor, finely grind almonds and mix with soy flour, sweetener, and baking powder.
3. In separate bowl, on medium speed, mix whole egg, butter, egg yolk, and vanilla. Mixture will not be smooth.
4. Fold in soy flour mixture with rubber spatula until combined.
5. Form 24 small balls with dough and place on ungreased baking sheet.
6. Using a fork, slightly flatten to silver dollar size.
7. Bake 8-10 mins and allow to cool on baking sheets before moving to wire rack.

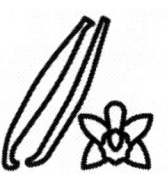

TIRAMISU CUPCAKES

Total Prep Time: 40 mins | Servings: 6
Nutrition Information:
Calories: 293 | Fat: 24 g | Carbs: 3 g
Protein: 5 g | Fiber: 11 g

What You'll Need:

- 3 Tbsp butter, unsalted
- 3 large whole eggs
- ¼ c sucralose sweetener
- 5 Tbsp xylitol sweetener
- 4 Tbsp vanilla extract
- ¼ c coconut flour, organic & high fiber
- ¼ tsp baking powder
- ¼ tsp salt
- 4 oz mascarpone
- 1 ¼ Tbsp instant coffee powder
- ½ c heavy cream
- ½ oz water

What You'll Do:

NOTE: This recipe uses both sucralose and xylitol sweetener to give a rounded sweetness.

Cupcakes:

1. Preheat oven to 375°F/190°C. Place liners in muffin tin and set aside.
2. With an electric mixer, blend sucralose sweetener and butter until fluffy- about 2 mins.
3. Add eggs, 1 tsp vanilla, baking powder, salt, and coconut flour, blending until smooth. Divide batter between 6 muffin cups.
4. Bake for about 15 mins.
5. Let rest in pan for 5 mins before removing to place on cooling rack.

Soaking syrup:

1. Combine 1 tsp instant coffee, 1 ½ Tbsp water, 2 Tbsp xylitol, and 2 tsp vanilla.
2. Poke cupcakes with toothpick and pour soaking syrup over each one.

Mascarpone Frosting:

1. Blend mascarpone cheese, ¼ instant coffee, 1 tsp vanilla, and 3 Tbsp xylitol until smooth.
2. In separate bowl, whip heavy cream until stiff peaks form.
3. Fold mascarpone cheese mixture into whipped cream until combined.
4. Place mixture in decorator/pastry bag with a fancy tip (if desired) and pipe onto cooled cupcakes- or you can just spread frosting onto cupcakes if you prefer.
5. Serve at room temp, dusted with cocoa powder. May be kept in fridge overnight in airtight container, if desired.

Low Carb Snack Recipes

BLACKBERRY-COCONUT FAT BOMBS

> *Total Prep Time: 10 mins | Servings: 16 bite-size squares*
> *Nutrition Information:*
> *Calories: 170 | Fat: 18 g*
> *Carbs: 3 g | Protein: 1 g*

What You'll Need:

- 1 c coconut butter
- 1 c coconut oil
- ½ c blackberries, strawberries, or raspberries
- ½ tsp sweetener, more to taste
- ½ tsp vanilla extract (or ¼ tsp vanilla powder)
- 1 Tbsp lemon juice

What You'll Do:

1. Place coconut oil & butter (& if frozen, berries) in pot. Heat until just combined on medium heat. If using fresh berries, do not add them yet.
2. Place oil mixture and other ingredients into blender and blend. You must ensure that oil mixture is not too hot, otherwise separation will occur.
3. Using parchment paper, line square pan and pour mixture in.
4. Place in fridge for an hour or until mixture has hardened.
5. Cut into squares and enjoy.
6. Store in fridge, covered.

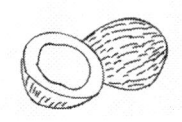

PIZZA BITES

> *Total Prep Time: 25 mins | Servings: 28*
> *Nutrition Information:*
> *Calories: 60 | Fat: 5 g*
> *Carbs: 1 | Protein: 2.5 g*

What You'll Need:

- ½ c almond flour
- ½ c parmesan cheese, grated
- ½ tsp each basil and garlic powder
- ¼ tsp each salt, oregano, and thyme
- ¼ c coconut flour
- 2 tsp baking powder
- 4-oz mozzarella, shredded
- 2 to 3 oz chopped pepperoni
- 4 Tbsp butter, room temp
- 2 large eggs
- ½ c sour cream
- Other Ingredients (as desired)
- ¼ c olives, chopped
- ½ bell pepper or small onion, chopped and sautéed
- 4 oz mushrooms, chopped and sautéed
- If you wish, omit basil, oregano, and thyme
- and use 1 tsp Italian seasoning instead

What You'll Do:

1. Preheat oven to 350°F/176°C. Place parchment paper on 2 pans and set aside.
2. In a medium-size bowl, add dry ingredients and blend.
3. Add the rest of the ingredients and mix until well blended with a spatula or wooden spoon.
4. Use a small scoop for smaller bites and a medium scoop for larger bites to measure dough onto pans and place 3 inches apart.

5. Bake until brown, 15-20 mins.
6. Serve with pizza sauce or ranch dressing.

SALT & VINEGAR ZUCCHINI CHIPS

Total Prep Time: 12 hours 15 mins | Servings: 8
Nutrition Information:
Calories: 40 | Fat: 3 g
Carbs: 3 g | Protein: .7 g

What You'll Need:

- 2-3 medium zucchini, thinly sliced
- 2 Tbsp olive oil, sunflower oil, or avocado oil
- 2 Tbsp white balsamic vinegar
- 2 tsp sea salt

What You'll Do:

1. Slice zucchini thin.
2. Combine oil and vinegar in a separate bowl.
3. Place zucchini in bowl with oil & vinegar and toss until covered.
4. Place zucchini in even layers in food dehydrator and sprinkle with sea salt. Depending upon how thin your zucchini is and your dehydrator, the time will vary- from 8 to 14 hours.
5. These can be done in your oven if you do not have a food dehydrator.
6. Using parchment paper, line baking sheet and place zucchini in an even layer.
7. Bake at 200°F/93°C for 2-3 hours, flipping chips over halfway through cook time.
8. Must be stored in a container with a tight seal.

CHOCOLATE QUINOA BITES

Total Prep Time: 10 mins | Servings: 12
Nutrition Facts
Calories: 175 | Fat: 13 g
Carbs: 13 g | Protein: 3 g

What You'll Need:

- ¼ c coconut oil
- ¼ c maple syrup
- 1/3 c unsweetened cocoa powder
- ½ c nut/seed butter of choice
- ½ c quinoa, cooked
- ½ c quinoa flakes
- ½ c coconut flakes
- Sea salt for sprinkling, if desired

What You'll Do:

1. Line baking sheet with parchment paper.
2. Melt coconut oil, syrup, and cocoa powder together in small saucepan over medium heat, whisking until combined.
3. Add almond butter. Blend until smooth.
4. Remove from heat and fold in coconut flakes, quinoa, and quinoa flakes.
5. Using a cookie scoop, drop onto prepared baking sheet, and sprinkle with sea salt (if desired) and place in freezer for about 30 minutes to set.
6. For best results, store in freezer in airtight container- but can be kept in fridge, if you want a softer consistency.

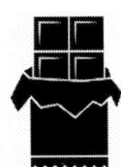

PEPPER NACHOS

> *Total Prep Time: 20 mins | Servings: 6*
> *Nutrition Information:*
> *Calories: 351 | Cholesterol: 96 mg | Fat: 21 g*
> *Carbs: 6 g | Protein: 28 g*

What You'll Need:

- 1 tsp each garlic powder, cumin, and paprika
- 1 Tbsp chili powder
- ½ tsp each salt, pepper, and oregano
- ¼ tsp red pepper flakes (more if you want it hotter)
- 1 lb ground beef
- 1 lb mini peppers, halved & seeded
- 1 ½ c cheddar cheese, shredded
- ½ c tomato, chopped
- Other toppings, such as avocado, olives, chopped jalapenos, sour cream, etc.

What You'll Do:

1. Combine all spices in separate bowl and set aside.
2. Brown beef in skillet over medium heat- about 7-10 mins. Add spice mixture and sauté until combined.
3. Preheat oven to 400°F/204°C and line baking sheet with parchment paper or foil.
4. Arrange peppers close together, cut side up, in a single layer.
5. Sprinkle with ground beef and shredded cheese, making sure each pepper has some on it.
6. Bake 5-10 mins.
7. Take out of oven and add extra toppings as desired.

Low Carb Smoothie Recipes

CHOCOLATE-AVOCADO SMOOTHIE

Prep Time: 5 mins | Servings: 1
Nutrition Information:
Calories: 582 | Cholesterol: 81 mg
Carbs: 30 g | Protein: 9 g

What You'll Need:

- Avocado, peel & remove pit
- ½ c heavy cream (decrease calorie count by substituting milk)
- 1 Tbsp dark cocoa powder
- 3 tsp Splenda (or preferred sweetener)
- 1 c water

What You'll Do:

1. Place all ingredients in blender and blend until smooth.
2. Serve cold.

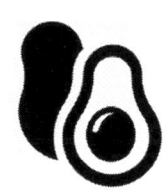

VERY BERRY SMOOTHIE

Prep Time: 5 mins | Servings: 1
Nutrition Information:
Calories: 129 | Fat: 3 g | Cholesterol: 7 mg
Carbs: 18 g | Protein: 7 g

What You'll Need:

- ½ c unsweetened almond milk
- ½ c low-fat yogurt
- ½ cup frozen berry mix (blackberries, raspberries, strawberries, blueberries)
- 1 tsp sweetener of choice

What You'll Do:

1. Place all ingredients in blender and blend until smooth.
2. Serve cold.

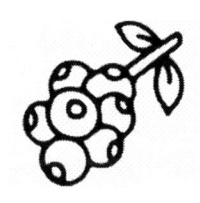

CHOCOLATE PEANUT BUTTER SMOOTHIE

Prep Time: 5 mins | Servings: 1
Nutrition Information:
Calories: 457 | Total Fat: 32 g | Cholesterol: 85 mg
Total Carbs: 20 g | Protein: 25 g

What You'll Need:

- 1 c almond milk, unsweetened
- 2 c ice
- 2 Tbsp natural peanut butter, unsweetened
- 2 Tbsp cocoa powder, unsweetened
- 1 scoop vanilla flavored protein powder
- 2 Tbsp heavy whipping cream
- ¼ tsp vanilla extract
- Sweetener, to taste (optional)

What You'll Do:

1. Place almond milk, whipping cream, peanut butter, vanilla extract, cocoa powder, protein powder, and sweetener into blender.
2. Blend until smooth and serve cold.

COFFEE SMOOTHIE

> *Prep Time: 5 mins | Servings: 1*
> *Nutrition Information:*
> *Calories: 294 | Fat: 19 g | Cholesterol: 91 mg*
> *Carbs: 10 g | Protein: 23 g*

What You'll Need:

- 16 oz vanilla flavored almond milk, unsweetened
- 1 tsp instant coffee
- 1 Tbsp ground flax seed
- 2 Tbsp cream cheese
- 1 scoop protein powder

What You'll Do:

1. Place all ingredients in blender and blend until smooth.
2. Serve immediately.

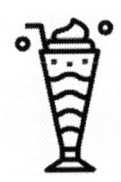

AVOCADO/SPINACH/STRAWBERRY SMOOTHIE

Prep Time: 5 mins | Servings: 1
Nutrition Information:
Calories: 296 | Fat: 22 g | Cholesterol 0 mg
Carbs: 26 g | Protein: 5 g

What You'll Need:

- 1 medium avocado
- ½ c frozen sliced strawberries
- 4 oz grape juice
- ½ cup fresh spinach

What You'll Do:

1. Place all ingredients in blender and blend until smooth.

Bonus: 10 Ways to Lose Weight Fast

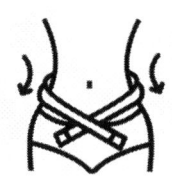

These days, it seems like everywhere you look, there's someone that's looking for the secret to lose weight fast. While there's no magical solution, the best thing to do is to stop the yo-yo dieting and commit to a true lifestyle change- such as the low-carb lifestyle. After all, most diets require you to restrict yourself and are not realistic solutions. In this section, we'll outline 10 ways that you can jump start weight loss as you begin your journey.

Begin Your Day with Warm Lemon Water

Lemon water will get your digestive system moving and help flush out toxins. You'll also want to commit to drinking at least 8 glasses of water every day. This will help speed up your metabolism and curb your hunger.

Get at least 30 mins of Physical Activity Daily

Exercising will not only help you lose weight, but also help you maintain your weight. Plus, when you work up a sweat, your body is able to fight off a variety of health conditions/disease- and your mood is improved. Just because you're committing to working out doesn't mean that you're stuck to the gym. There are lots of ways that you can burn calories. Find a few things you enjoy and start practicing them. You might want to consider alternating them as well, so you don't get burnt out.

Be Sure to Get Your Fiber

Foods that are rich in fiber keep you feeling fuller longer. This means you won't eat as much. In addition, fiber aids in digestion and lowers your blood sugar and cholesterol.

Consume Healthy Protein Sources at Every Meal

Protein also keeps you feeling fuller longer, as well as promoting muscle growth and repair. However, you must make sure that you're consuming clean proteins, such as pastured eggs, organic chicken, wild salmon, or grass-fed beef. If you're a vegan, consider adding healthy grains/beans and flax, hemp, and chia seeds.

Pay Attention to What You're Eating

Make sure that you pay attention to what you're eating and what is actually going to give you nourishment. If there's not a good reason behind eating something, you probably shouldn't be eating it. Don't eat while you're distracted- and take it slow because it takes about 20 mins from the time you begin your meal for your brain to realize that your stomach is full.

Choose Healthy Snacks

Choosing healthy snacks is just as important as choosing healthy meals because they help balance your blood sugar and energy levels. You shouldn't worry about snacks labeled diet/low fat/fat free. The idea is to choose fresh, whole foods.

Discover Healthy Alternatives to Your Favorite Treats

If there is something that you really enjoy, don't eliminate it from your diet. Instead, give yourself permission to splurge once a week- but take the time to make it yourself. This way, you have control of what goes into it. Unfortunately, it's easy to find unhealthy recipes, so it will take a little effort to find some healthier alternatives.

Learn to Manage Your Stress

Cortisol, which is the hormone that is related to stress, results in belly fat, food cravings, and increased appetite. Take the time to de-stress when you feel it coming on. This can be by writing in a journal, practicing yoga/meditation, practicing deep breathing exercises, and many other activities. Everyone is faced with stress. The key is learning the best way for you to deal with it.

Kick Those Bad Habits

Of course, reaching that ideal, healthy lifestyle is not just about changing your eating habits. There are many other things that could be sabotaging your life: smoking, drinking too much soda or alcohol, not getting enough sleep, and much more. Take an inventory of your daily habits and start changing those that you think are holding you back. This is going to be difficult, so take baby steps.

Make a Plan to be Successful

Every successful person started with a plan in place to encourage that success. If you don't plan to succeed, then you're planning to fail. If you will make an effort to remove all unhealthy foods from you kitchen and you start making meal prep a priority, you'll find that it's easier to be committed to your goals.

While it's true that dieting will jumpstart your weight loss journey, you have to make an effort to lose and maintain it. The best thing to do is to make some changes in your lifestyle and soon, you'll find that the extra weight is gone and you're feeling much better in all aspects: physically, mentally, and emotionally. If you do slip back into your old habits, don't beat yourself up- just reaffirm your commitment to changing your life. Good luck!

Intermittent Fasting

Intermittent Fasting and How it Works

Intermittent Fasting (IF) is currently a popular health trend and weight loss measure which involves alternating between brief periods of fasting, with either no food or substantialcalorie reduction, and periods of unrestricted eating. Research has shown that intermittent fasting is not only effective for weight loss but also changes body composition through loss of fat mass and improves metabolic health. Fasting over short periods reduces calorie intake and belly fat and optimizes certain hormones involved in weight control, subject of course to not over indulging during eating periods.

No, it is not a means of starvation. Starvation is not controlled, and it is not voluntary, for the most part. Starvation can therefore be described as involuntary and involves a total absence of food over an extended period. It causes suffering and may prove fatal. Fasting, in contrast, involves a voluntary denying of food, maybe for health or spiritual reasons. Fasters are not underweight, and therefore have sufficient stored body fat to support the body, eliminating suffering and the risk of death. While fasting, decisions can be made depending on the circumstances, to maintain health and wellbeing while restricting food intake.

Strength training during IF is recommended to effectively retain muscle while burning fat. It is basically impossible to gain muscle and lose fat at the same time. More calories must be burnt than are consumed to lose fat, therefore a net calorie deficit is necessary. To build muscle, more calories are needed than are burnt, and so a net calorie surplus is necessary. By cycling calorie and carbohydrate intake, more calories and carbs are consumed on training days and less calories and carbs on resting days. In this way the calories fuel the body during strength training, leaving a calorie deficit on days on which no training is done. In this way muscle is built during training and fat is burnt on rest days.

Hydration while fasting is important. Of course, staying hydrated is always important but more so when food intake is reduced during Intermittent Fasting, this is because food is responsible for about a fifth of daily water consumption. Anyone who has experienced the dehydration headache will know the struggle! Drinking can also overcome hunger while fasting, but you should know what to drink:

Mineral water or any water, really, is calorie free and permitted when fasting. The reason mineral water is preferred is because it contains minerals which assist electrolyte and mineral imbalance restoration.

Coffee is not only allowed but it is an appetite suppressant and may in fact reduce insulin sensitivity and support fat burning over time. But too much is bad. Moderation is key and the recommended daily intake is just over two cups of brewed coffee.

Apple cider vinegar is also free of calories and therefore allowed. An added benefit is that it aids digestion and helps to lower blood sugar levels.

Certain natural sweeteners are permitted for those who can't do without the sweetness but be mindful of going organic and stay away from any with negative side effects.

Coconut oil/other oils affect insulin and blood glucose very little but be mindful that fats are very high in calories.

Butter, like coconut oil, affects insulin very little if at all, and is also extremely high in calories.

Almond milk **without** added sugar or fortified with extra protein, is low in calories and carbs, and a good option for vegans.

Bear in mind these important aspects of losing weight through Intermittent Fasting:

- ✓ *Calories* still matter, which means it is important to eat normally during the eating windows rather than to over indulge.

- ✓ *Consistency* is imperative. This is not a crash diet. Commitment over time is required for it to be successful.

- ✓ *Food Quality* goes hand in hand with a healthy diet. Make healthy choices.

- ✓ *Patience* also goes hand in hand with consistency. Adaptation to the diet is necessary and this will only happen if the meal schedule is adhered to over time.

A popular method is to fast either on alternate days, during a set time, or over a specific frequency per week for an entire day.

- ✓ *Alternate-day fasting* involves fluctuating between unrestricted eating days and days where only one meal is taken which provides 25% of the required daily calories. In this instance, for example, fasting days would be Monday, Wednesday and Friday. On Tuesday, Thursday and weekends, no food restrictions apply.

- ✓ *Time-restricted feeding* designates a certain time frame for fasting, for example, meals are unrestricted from 11am to 6pm, and the rest of the day is spent fasting.

- ✓ *Whole-day fasting* involves complete fasting or up to 25% of daily calorie needs on one or two days per week and no food restriction on the other days. For example, the 5:2 diet approach does not restrict food for five days while the remaining two days restricts calories to 400 to 500 per day.

Let's look more in depth at how IF positively affects hormones. We now know that energy is stored in body fat as calories. When the body is not fed regularly, changes in metabolism and hormones occurs to make stored energy more accessible. These changes include:

- ✓ *Insulin* decreases substantially when fasting, and lower levels of insulin help to burn fat;
- ✓ *Noradrenaline* is released by the nervous system to break fat down into free fatty acids in the fat cells, to be used for energy.

- ✓ *Human Growth Hormone (HGH)* skyrockets during fasting by up to five times. This hormone aids fat loss and muscle gain.

How would Intermittent Fasting assist in reducing calories and losing weight? Of course a lower calorie intake is probably the biggest reason. IF has been found to reduce body weight by an average of 0.25kg per week. Weight loss of up to 8% was measured over three to twenty-four weeks. Waist circumference is reduced by between 4 and 7% which indicates loss of belly fat. Intermittent Fasting may lead to retention of muscle while dieting. Muscle loss is usually a negative side effect accompanying the burning of fat during weight loss. Intermittent Fasting is an easier way to eat healthier, because it allows for less than 3 meals per day which means fewer opportunities to over indulge on unhealthy food.

These are the benefits of Intermittent Fasting for weight loss:

- ✓ *Lower insulin levels* boost adiponectin levels, restoring insulin sensitivity and thereby preventing diabetes and weight gain. Lowered insulin also tells the body to burn stored fat rather than glucose.

- ✓ *Boosts metabolism*, which kickstarts the body to burn more calories throughout the day, including while at rest. Adrenaline and noradrenaline levels increase during fasting, and these hormones help to free energy stored in body fat.

- ✓ *Ketosis* is a fat burning state in which the body, once drained of glucose, burns the fat reserves to access energy to fuel activity and brain power. Ketosis reduces inflammation and improves blood chemistry. Full ketosis usually involves limiting carbohydrates drastically and careful planning, but this is fast tracked through IF.

- ✓ *Reduces inflammation*, which boots longevity, reduces risk of certain illnesses and chronic diseases and is key to weight loss.

The accepted rule is to remain in a fasting state by consuming less than 50 calories while fasting. This makes it easier to accept not eating during this time, as coffee, green tea and water are all allowed or encouraged. In fact, hydration is vital during fasting. In fact, many find the want to increase their water intake when they get into Intermittent Fasting.

It is important to consult a medical professional before embarking on any dietary plan. *Intermittent Fasting is not recommended for:*

- ✓ Pregnant and breastfeeding women
- ✓ Anyone who tends to suffer from eating disorders, such as anorexia or bulimia nervosa, or partakes in unhealthy self-restriction
- ✓ Persons on medications that require food intake
- ✓ People in active growth stage, such as in adolescents

Various methods of Intermittent Fasting have been devised and their efficacy depends highly on the individual. We will briefly explain two of the preferred types of IF: the 16:8 method and the 5:2 method, and which method may be best.

THE 16:8 METHOD

Leangains protocol or the 16:8 Method was popularized by Martin Berkhan, a fitness expert. Participants fast for 14 to 16 hours every day, allowing a daily eating window of between 8 and 10 hours during which 2 or 3 meals can be eaten. This method of IF is as simple as skipping breakfast and fasting after the evening meal. In this way fasting for 16 hours can be achieved fairly easily in men, and 14 to 15 hours in women.

THE 5:2 METHOD

This IF involves eating normally for 5 days and restricting calories to between 500 and 600 on the remaining two days. Also known as the Fast diet, it was popularized by Michael Mosley, a British journalist and doctor.

Women should eat 500 calories and men 600 calories on the two fasting days, over two small meals of 250/300 calories each, while consuming normal meals on every other day.

Which method is best?

Intermittent fasting is not right for everyone and should only be used for those who find the methods useful. It is thought that men might find it more beneficial than women. Whatever the case, it is certainly not the right choice for individuals prone to eating disorders.

The 16:8 method may not be best for those who like their breakfasts in the mornings. For habitual breakfast skippers, however, this method is more or less already an instinctive way of eating.

Individuals who prefer smaller meals may do well with the 5:2 method, in the knowledge that they will not suffer on restricted calories for 2 days in the week.

As with any fasting diet, the importance lies in eating high quality, healthy food during the eating windows, and not consuming high volumes of empty calories. Fasting is not healthy for individuals suffering certain health issues or diseases and illnesses, and care should always be taken to consult a medical professional before embarking on Intermittent Fasting diets.

Mediterranean Diet

Mediterranean Diet Cookbook

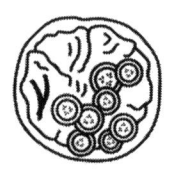

As one of the world's most popular diets today, the Mediterranean diet doesn't use a strict meal plan. Instead, it focuses on whole foods and exercise. In this cookbook, we are going to give you a nice introduction and some scrumptious recipes you can use to live the Mediterranean lifestyle.

What is the Mediterranean Diet?

The countries surrounding the Mediterranean Sea have very similar eating patterns, and that is what the Mediterranean diet is based off of. You will not find a set bunch of rules, either (although there are some guidelines). The meals prepared for this diet use whole fruits, vegetables, grains, legumes, and olive oils, as well as other healthy fats. You will find that lean proteins, like chicken and pork, will be used regularly, as will fish. You will also use some red meat, but very little compared to the Western diet. You will be able to drink in moderation.

This diet is designed to help reduce your cholesterol, lower heart disease risks, and help you live an all-around healthier and longer life.

How to Get Started

Getting started with the idea that you should base your diet around the healthy habits of the population that lives around the Mediterranean, there are a few ideas that you may want to consider:

- Always focus on whole foods. Eliminate processed foods as much as possible
- Limit your red meat intake. You don't have to cut red meat out of your diet completely, but limiting yourself to a couple of times a month is a great idea.
- Cook with olive oil whenever you can. Olive oil is the main fat source in the Mediterranean, and it is a healthy fat.
- Reduce your dairy consumption. Limit the amount of cheese and milk-based products. Use yogurt as a substitute whenever you can.
- Get rid of refined grains. Replace your pasta and rice with items like quinoa and bulgur. Whole grains are a big part of the food of the Mediterranean, because they are rich in fiber and vitamin B.
- Nuts are great snacks. They are rich in omega fatty acids, protein and fiber. Snacking on nuts with fruits or vegetables will help you stay full longer.
- Now that you are armed with some great tips, it is time to share with you some great recipe options that will help you build a healthier, happier, and longer life.

RECIPES

Breakfast

AVOCADO TOAST CAPRESE STYLE

Servings: 2

Ingredients

- 2 pcs. whole-wheat/multigrain bread
- 8 halved grape tomatoes
- 2 oz. fresh mozzarella balls (approx. 12)
- Basil leaves, freshly torn
- 2 tbsp. balsamic vinegar or glaze
- Salt & pepper

Directions

1. Toast the bread to your preferred level of brown. As you are toasting the bread, cut and peel the avocado and put into a small bowl. Then mash until you reach your desired consistency. Add salt and pepper to taste.
2. Remove the toast from the toaster and spread the avocado on each slice. Once this is done, place the grape tomatoes, mozzarella, and basil over each slice.
3. Drizzle with balsamic vinegar and serve.

Nutritional Facts
Calories: 649 | Carbs: 86.4g | Fat: 24.6g | Protein: 23.9g

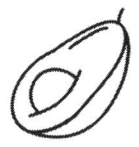

FRITTATA W/ ASPARAGUS, MUSHROOM, & GOAT CHEESE

Servings: 4

Ingredients

- 2 eggs
- 1 tsp. water or milk
- Kosher salt, 1 pinch
- Cooking spray (or 1 tbsp. butter)
- 2 or 3 sliced mushrooms
- 4-5 trimmed, cut asparagus spears
- 1 tbsp. green onion, chopped
- 2 tbsp. goat cheese

Directions

1. Set your oven to broil and let it begin the preheating process.
2. Lightly coat a medium-sized (7 - 8") frying pan with cooking spray. Place on a medium heat and let warm. Once it is heated a little, add mushrooms and sauté until they are slightly soft. Then, add in the asparagus. Cook the asparagus and mushrooms for a few more minutes.
3. Break the eggs into a small bowl and whisk with the teaspoon of water or milk and a pinch of kosher salt. Continue until the eggs have a nice froth, and the whites and yolk are completely combined.
4. Pour the egg mixture over the asparagus and mushroom mixture. Top with the goat cheese and green onions. Let cook until the edges begin to brown and pull away from the pan. Lift the eggs gently, tilting the pan to allow for any uncooked egg mixture to begin to cool.
5. Take a pan and move to the oven. Let the frittata grill for a few minutes. This will finish the cooking process and allow the eggs to puff. When removed from the oven, sprinkle a little more cheese on top. Slice into wedges and serve.

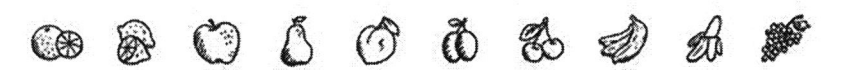

Nutritional Facts
Calories: 274 | Carbs: 10g | Fat: 18g | Protein: 15g

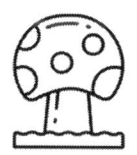

POACHED EGG WITH GREENS & WHITE BEANS

Servings: 4

Ingredients

- 3 tbsp. olive oil (divided into individual tbsp.)
- 15 oz. can of cannellini beans, drained and rinsed
- 1 tsp. kosher salt
- 2 tsp. za'atar
- 1 med. bunch, Swiss chard, thinly sliced & stems removed
- 2 garlic cloves, minced
- ¼ tsp. crushed red pepper flakes
- 1 tbsp. lemon juice, freshly squeezed

Directions

1. Crack each egg into individual cups. Fill the crockpot with water and a teaspoon of vinegar. Let it begin to simmer. Stir the water until there is a whirlpool effect and slowly tip one egg at a time into the center. Cook each egg for 3-4 minutes and then remove gently to a paper towel with a slotted spoon.
2. Now heat 2 tbsp of oil in the frying pan on medium heat until the oil is hot. Add a can of drained and rinsed cannellini beans. Make sure the beans are spread in an even layer and let cook until the cannellini beans are slightly brown on the bottom.
3. Add ½ tsp. of salt and 1 tsp. of za'atar and stir. Then spread the beans back out in an even layer and cook until the beans are blistered on the side.
4. Add the remaining oil to the pan, as well as the chard. Now sprinkle in the remaining salt, the za'atar, garlic, and pepper flakes. Cook until the chard has wilted down. Then remove from the pan and add the lemon juice. Divide the mixture into serving bowls and top with poached egg and, if desired, more crushed pepper flakes.

Nutritional Facts
Calories: 301 | Carbs: 26.5g | Fat: 15.5g | Protein: 15.5g

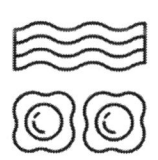

START YOUR MORNING RIGHT GRAIN SALAD

Servings: 8

Ingredients

- 1 cup oats, steel-cut
- 1 cup quinoa, dry golden
- ½ cup millet, dry
- 3 tbsp. olive oil
- ¾ tsp. salt
- 1 pc. fresh ginger, peeled and cut into discs
- 2 lrg. Lemons, zest and juice
- ½ cup maple syrup
- 1 cup yogurt, Greek
- ¼ tsp. nutmeg
- 2 cups hazelnuts, toasted and chopped
- 2 cups blueberries, fresh

Directions

1. Pour and mix the oats, millet, and quinoa into a fine-mesh strainer and wash under cool running water for a minute. Then, set aside to drain.
2. Over medium-high heat, heat 1 tbsp. of olive oil in a saucepan. Add the rinsed grains and cook for a few minutes, until they begin to smell toasted. Now, add 4 ½ cups of water, along with ¾ tsp. of salt, the ginger, and the zest of 1 lemon.
3. Bring mixture to a boil, cover with a lid, and turn down heat. Let simmer for 20 minutes. Turn off heat and remove. Leave standing for 5 minutes. Then, remove the lid and use a fork to fluff the mixture. Take out the ginger coins. Now, take the mixture and spread it out over a baking sheet. Leave to cool for about 30 minutes. Once it has cooled, spoon into large bowl and mix in the zest of the lemon.
4. Combine in medium-sized bowl with 2 tbsp. of olive oil and the juice of two lemons. Whisk until emulsified. Add in maple syrup, yogurt, and nutmeg, and whisk until completely combined. Then, pour over the grain mixture and stir until coated. Add in toasted hazelnuts and blueberries. Taste and add seasonings as desired.
5. Let sit in the refrigerator overnight and enjoy.

Nutritional Facts
Calories: 353 | Carbs: 38.0g | Fat: 20.1g | Protein: 9.3g

EASY MUESLI

Servings: 8

Ingredients

- 3 ½ cups oats, rolled
- ½ cup wheat bran
- ½ tsp. salt, kosher
- ½ tsp. cinnamon, ground
- ½ cup almonds, sliced
- ¼ cup pecans, chopped
- ¼ cup pepitas
- ½ cup coconut flakes, unsweetened
- ¼ cup apricots, dried, chopped
- ¼ cup cherries, dried

Directions

1. Start by toasting the grains, seeds, and nuts. Preheat oven to 350° F and make sure the two racks are evenly distributed. Place the grains on one baking sheet with the salt and cinnamon. Evenly spread nuts and seeds on another baking sheet. Place both baking sheets in the oven and bake until you can smell the nuts. This usually takes 10 – 12 minutes.
2. Remove baking sheet with the nuts and allow to cool. Pull the grain sheet out and add in the coconut and place back in oven. Bake for further five minutes, or until the coconut is lightly browned. Remove from the oven and allow to cool.
3. Add both baking sheets to large bowl, then toss in dried fruits and combine.
4. Place mixture in an airtight container that can be stored at room temperature for up to a month.

Nutritional Facts
Calories: 275 | Carbs: 36.4g | Fat: 13.0g | Protein: 8.5g

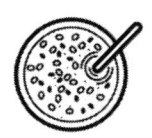

Meat

GRILLED BALSAMIC CHICKEN W/ OLIVE TAPENADE

Servings: 2

Ingredients

- 2 chicken breasts, boneless, skinless
- ¼ cup olive oil
- ¼ cup balsamic vinegar, golden
- ⅛ cup mustard, whole grain
- 1 ½ tbsp. balsamic vinegar
- 3 garlic cloves, minced

- Lemon juice, ½ of one lemon
- ½ tbsp. rosemary, fresh
- ½ tbsp. thyme, fresh
- ½ tbsp. basil, fresh
- 1 tsp. salt, kosher
- ½ tsp. pepper, freshly ground
- Feta cheese, chunked

Tapenade

- 3 garlic cloves, minced
- ¼ cup olive oil
- ½ cup sun-dried tomatoes, drained and chopped
- 4 oz. jar green olives, drained and pitted

- 6 oz. jar kalamata olives, drained and pitted
- 1 small jar of capers, drained
- Lemon juice, fresh (whole lemon)
- 2 tsp. balsamic vinegar
- ½ tsp. pepper, freshly ground
- ⅓ cup parsley, fresh, chopped

Directions

Tapenade Directions

1. Place the garlic and olive oil into the food processor and run it on high until everything is completely combined. Open the lid and scrape down the sides, then add sun-dried tomatoes and capers. Run through the processor until tomatoes are chopped.
2. Now, add olives and pulse until olives are coarsely chopped. Add in lemon juice, vinegar, pepper, parsley, and remaining capers. Stir until mixed thoroughly.

Balsamic Chicken Directions

1. Trim the chicken of any excess fat and place it in a freezer bag.
2. In a small bowl, combine the olive oil, vinegar, mustard, garlic, lemon juice, herbs, salt, and pepper. Whisk until all Ingredients are mixed well. Reserve half of the mixture and pour the rest into the freezer bag. Leave it to marinate for a minimum of 30 minutes (best if left overnight), turning occasionally.
3. Heat grill pan and drizzle olive oil into it. Then place the chicken breasts on the grill. Grill for 3 minutes on each side (depending on how thick the breast is, it may need less or more time to cook). This will give the nice grill marks. Then, lower heat and grill for another 5 minutes per side or until you have an internal temp of 165°F. While cooking the breasts, have a small bowl of the mixture near you so that you can baste the chicken with it.
4. Remove breasts to a plate and tent with foil for another 5 minutes to allow the juices to redistribute. Then, serve with tapenade and a sprinkle of feta cheese. Finish off with a drizzle of the reserved marinade over the top.

Nutritional Facts
Calories: 261.2 | Carbs: 3.8g | Fat: 15.2g | Protein: 26.1g

PORK SCALOPPINI W/ LEMON AND CAPERS

Servings: 4

Ingredients

- 4 pork chops, thin, boneless
- 8 sage leaves, fresh
- ¼ cup flour, all-purpose
- Kosher salt (for taste)
- Pepper (for taste)
- 4 tbsp. butter
- 1 tbsp. vegetable oil
- ½ cup wine, white
- ¼ cup capers, drained
- 1 cup stock, chicken
- Lemon juice, fresh (2 lemons)
- 1 lemon, sliced thinly
- 2 tbsp. parsley, flat-leaf, chopped

Directions

1. Pound the pork chops until they are ¼ inch thick. Then, press two sage leaves per chop into the meat.

2. Combine flour, salt, and pepper in a shallow bowl. Coat the pork chops in the flour, being careful not to dislodge the sage leaves. Carefully remove excess flour.

3. Heat the skillet over medium heat and melt 1 tbsp. of butter with ½ tbsp. of the oil. Place two of the pork chops into the heated skillet and cook for about 4 minutes per side. Remove and set aside. Add another tbsp. of butter, the remaining oil and repeat the process with the last 2 chops.

4. Carefully wipe out the skillet to get rid of most of the crispy bits. Then, replace on heat and melt another tablespoon of butter in skillet. Once it is melted, add in the wine and capers. Cook this down until it is reduced by half. Then, add in the stock, lemon juice, and some of the lemon slices. Bring to a boil and then add the rest of the butter into the skillet. Let simmer until the sauce thickens. Then, add chops back into skillet. Let them heat up in the sauce. Serve topped with chopped parsley.

Nutritional Facts
Calories: 415 | Carbs: 14g | Fat: 24g | Protein: 31g

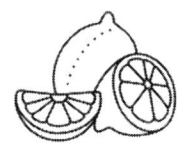

GREEK TURKEY BURGERS

Servings: 4

Ingredients

- 1 lb. turkey, ground
- ½ cup spinach, fresh, chopped
- ⅓ cup sun-dried tomatoes, chopped
- ¼ cup red onion, minced
- ¼ cup feta, crumbled
- 2 garlic cloves, minced
- 1 egg, whisked
- 1 tbsp. olive oil
- 1 tsp. oregano, dried
- ½ tsp. salt, kosher
- ½ tsp. pepper, freshly ground
- 4 whole-wheat buns
- Lettuce leaves, Bibb
- Red onion, sliced

Tzatziki Ingredients

- ½ cucumber, grated, skin and seeds removed
- ¾ cup Greek yogurt, low-fat
- 2 garlic cloves, minced
- 1 tbsp. red wine vinegar
- 1 tbsp. dill, fresh, minced
- Pinch of kosher salt and pepper

Directions

1. Put the ground turkey, spinach, sun-dried tomatoes, red onion and feta in a large bowl. Then, combine garlic, egg, olive oil, oregano, salt, and pepper in small bowl and whisk until thoroughly emulsified. Pour into large bowl with turkey. Mix with your hands and, when completely mixed, divide into four patties. Place on parchment paper that has been laid over a cutting board. Then, refrigerate for at least 30 minutes (overnight is great, as well).

2. Make the tzatziki sauce. Start by grating the cucumber. Then, place in a paper towel and squeeze to remove the water. Now, you can place it in a small bowl. Add the yogurt, vinegar, dill, garlic, salt, and pepper. Mix until completely combined. Cover the bowl and let stand in refrigerator for at least 30 minutes.

3. Spray some cooking spray on a grill pan, and heat it over a medium heat
4. Place turkey burgers on grill pan and cook for about 5 minutes per side. Remove when cooked through and let rest for a minute.
5. Spread tzatziki on the buns and use the red onion, lettuce, and garnishes for the burger.

Nutritional Facts
Calories: 350 | Carbs: 10g | Fat: 7g | Protein: 54g

POMEGRANATE CITRUS GLAZED DUCK BREAST

Servings: 4

Ingredients

- 2 duck breasts
- Kosher salt and freshly ground black pepper
- 2 tbsp. pomegranate molasses
- 2 tbsp. white vermouth
- 1 lrg. orange, juiced
- 1 tbsp. honey
- 1 cinnamon stick
- 4 cloves, whole
- 1/8 tsp. cardamom

Directions

1. Preheat oven to 400° F. Then, on a cutting board, place duck breast fat side up. Use your paring knife to crosshatch the fat. Sprinkle with salt and pepper. Then, place them fat side down into a cold skillet and set the heat to low. Cook them like this for about 12-15 minutes. This renders off the fat.
2. While the duck is on the stove, combine the molasses, vermouth, orange juice, honey, cinnamon, cloves, and cardamom together in a small saucepan. Bring this up to a simmer and let simmer for about five minutes. Turn off the heat and set to the side.
3. Once the fat is rendered, drain it from skillet. Save and use later. Now, return duck breasts to pan, fat side up this time. Brush it with the pomegranate syrup you made earlier. Put pan in oven for roughly 5 – 7 minutes.
4. Once the duck is cooked and the temp reads 160°F, remove it from oven and place on a cutting board. Tent with foil to let rest, but not before you brush it again with the molasses syrup.

> Nutritional Facts
> Calories: 322 | Carbs: 28.2g | Fat: 7.2g | Protein: 33.3g

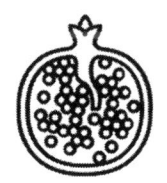

SKEWERED BEEF W/ GARLIC WHITE BEAN SAUCE

Servings: 16

Ingredients

- 1 lb. sirloin, boneless, cut 1" thick
- ½ tsp. garlic powder

Garlic White Bean Dip

- 1 can cannellini beans, drained and rinsed
- 2 tbsp. water
- 1 tbsp. balsamic vinegar
- ½ tsp. black pepper, freshly ground
- ¼ tsp paprika, smoked
- 3 tbsp. olive oil, extra virgin
- 1 clove garlic, chopped
- ½ tsp. salt
- ½ tsp. paprika, smoked

Directions

1. Start by making the dip. Place the beans, water, vinegar, 1 tbsp. of olive oil, garlic, and salt into the food processor. Process until smooth. Remove ½ of the dip, sprinkle with paprika, and drizzle 1 tsp. olive oil over the top. Then, place the rest of the dip on top of that and repeat the garnish process. Cover and set aside.
2. Soak bamboo skewers in water for approximately 10 minutes. While this is soaking, cut the beef into ¼" thick slices. Then, thread the beef onto the skewers.
3. Now, combine the garlic, pepper, and paprika into a small bowl and mix until combined. Sprinkle this mixture evenly over the skewers.
4. Place skewers onto a baking sheet and set oven to broil. Broil the skewers until they are done. Then, serve with dip.

Nutritional Facts
Calories: 70 | Carbs: 4g | Fat: 3g | Protein: 8g

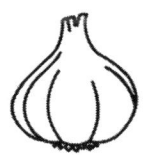

CHICKEN KEBABS

Servings: 6

Ingredients

- 1 lb. chicken breast, boneless, skinless
- ⅓ cup plain yogurt, Greek
- ¼ cup olive oil
- 4 lemons, juiced (1 zested)
- 5 garlic cloves, minced
- 2 tbsp. oregano, dried
- 1 tsp. kosher salt
- ½ tsp pepper, freshly ground
- 1 red onion, quartered 1" pcs.
- 1 zucchini, sliced ¼" pcs.
- 1 red bell pepper, cut into 1" pcs.

Directions

1. Cut chicken breasts into 1" pieces and place it in a freezer bag. Set aside.
2. Now, combine the Greek yogurt and olive oil into a medium bowl. Then, zest one whole lemon into the bowl and add the juice of lemon, as well. Now, add in the garlic, oregano, salt, pepper, and then mix well. Place half of the marinade into the freezer bag with the chicken. Cover and refrigerate the other half for use when cooking the chicken kebabs. Let chicken and marinade stand for at least 30 minutes.
3. Oil the grill pan (or grill). Soak your wooden skewers if using wood. Then, cut up the peppers, zucchini, and onion.
4. Now, it is time to assemble. Alternate vegetables and chicken until your skewer is full. Repeat the process until all your skewers are full.
5. Heat the grill pan (or grill) and then grill the skewers, using the remaining marinade to baste as you do so. Cook until the chicken juices run clear.

Nutritional Facts
Calories: 276 | Carbs: 8g | Fat: 6.1g | Protein: 45g

CHICKEN W/ TOMATO AND BALSAMIC SAUCE

Servings: 4

Ingredients

- 2 chicken breasts, boneless, skinless
- ½ tsp. salt
- ½ tsp. pepper, ground
- ¼ cup whole wheat flour, white
- 3 tbsp. olive oil, extra virgin
- ½ cup cherry tomatoes, halved
- 2 tbsp. shallots, sliced
- ¼ cup balsamic vinegar
- 1 cup chicken broth, low sodium
- 1 tbsp. garlic, minced
- 1 tbsp. fennel seeds, toasted and crushed
- 1 tbsp. butter

Directions

1. Cut each chicken breast in half horizontally. Then, lay on cutting board and place plastic wrap over the breasts. Pound the chicken breasts with the solid side of a meat tenderizer until ¼" thick. Remove the plastic wrap and sprinkle with 1⁄4tsp. each of salt and pepper on both sides. Then, place the flour in a shallow bowl. Dredge cutlets in flour, making sure to remove excess flour.

2. In a large skillet, heat 2 tbsp. of oil over a medium heat. Add two pieces of chicken, turning only once, and cook until evenly browned (about two to three minutes). Remove and repeat this process with the other two slices.

3. Once the chicken is removed, add the rest of the oil, tomatoes, and shallots to skillet. Cook until soft and then add the vinegar. Bring to a boil and scrape all the browned bits from the bottom of the skillet. Once the vinegar is reduced by half, add in the broth, fennel, and the rest of the salt and pepper. Cook while stirring continuously until the sauce is reduced by half. Then, remove from stove, add butter, and serve the sauce over the chicken.

Nutritional Facts
Calories: 294 | Carbs: 9g | Fat: 17g | Protein: 25g

MEDITERRANEAN SPAGHETTI SQUASH W/ TURKEY

Servings: 4

Ingredients

- 2 spaghetti squash
- 1 lb. ground turkey, lean
- 1 onion, diced
- 4 garlic cloves, minced
- 14 oz. canned diced tomatoes, Italian-style
- 2 cups mushrooms, sliced
- 6 oz. spinach
- 1 tsp. thyme
- 1 tsp. rosemary
- 1 tsp. basil, dried
- Salt and pepper
- 1 cup feta cheese

Directions

1. Preheat the oven to 400°F. Cut the spaghetti squash lengthwise and scoop out all the seeds. Sprinkle salt and pepper over the meat of the squash. Then, bake for 1 hour with the flesh side down.
2. Heat a skillet over a medium heat and add the turkey and onion into it. Cook until browned. Then, break the turkey up into little pieces and add garlic. Cook until the garlic is fragrant.
3. Next, add in the diced tomatoes (juice and all), mushrooms, spinach, thyme, rosemary, and dried basil. Bring this mixture up to a simmer and let it simmer while the spaghetti squash is baking. Taste and add seasonings if needed.
4. Once spaghetti squash is cooked, scoop out spaghetti squash and add to mixture.
5. Spray casserole dish and add the mixture into the dish. Top with feta and bake for 10 minutes.

Nutritional Facts
Calories: 540 | Carbs: 61g | Fat: 24g | Protein: 36g

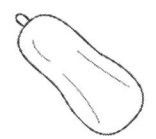

BONELESS PORK CHOPS W/ VEGETABLES

Servings: 4

Ingredients

- 8 pork chops, thin, boneless
- 1 sm. zucchini
- 1 sm. yellow squash
- 1 cup grape tomatoes, halved
- 1 tbsp. olive oil, extra-virgin
- ¼ tsp. kosher salt and pepper
- ¼ tsp. oregano
- 3 garlic cloves, sliced thin
- Cooking spray
- ¼ cup kalamata olives, pitted and sliced
- ¼ cup feta, crumbled
- Lemon juice fresh (half a lemon)
- 1 tsp. lemon rind, zested

Seasoning Ingredients

- ⅛ tsp. garlic powder
- ⅛ tsp. onion powder
- ⅛ tsp. lemon pepper
- ⅛ tsp. parsley flakes
- ⅛ tsp. coriander, ground
- ⅛ tsp. pepper
- ⅛ tsp. paprika
- ⅛ tsp. turmeric

Directions

1. In a small bowl, combine the Ingredients for the seasoning. Mix well. Then, preheat the oven to 450°F. Season the pork chops with the seasoning mixture.
2. Cut the zucchini and yellow squash into matchsticks (or use your mandolin). Then, in a bowl, toss the grape tomatoes with ½ tbsp. of oil, salt, pepper, and oregano. Spread the tomatoes onto a baking sheet and roast in the oven for 10 minutes, adding the garlic slices about halfway through. Once this is done, return mixture to the bowl and set to the side.
3. Reduce heat in the oven to 200°F. Then, heat skillet and add ½ tablespoon of oil, zucchini, squash, and salt. Sauté until tender and then add to tomatoes and place in oven to keep warm.

4. Cook the pork chops in batches over a medium heat for about 2 minutes per side. Then, remove vegetables from oven and add the lemon juice, lemon rind, and kalamata olives. Serve over the pork chops with feta cheese crumbled on top.

> *Nutritional Facts*
> Calories: 230 | Carbs: 9g | Fat: 9g | Protein: 28g

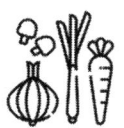

GARLIC STEAK W/ WARM SPINACH

Servings: 4

Ingredients

- 2 steaks, strip
- 4 ½ tsp. garlic, minced
- 1 cup red onion, thinly sliced
- 10 ½ oz. grape tomatoes, halved
- 10 oz. baby spinach, fresh

Directions

1. Take 2 ½ tsp. of minced garlic and press it evenly into the steaks. Cover them and let them stand in the refrigerator for 30 minutes.
2. Next, remove and place on a heated grill pan. Grill the steaks until the desired doneness, only turning occasionally.
3. Now, heat a large skillet and add onion and 2 tsp. of minced garlic. Cook until soft and garlic fragrant. Then, add tomatoes and kalamata olives. Cook these until soft, as well. Then, stir the spinach and take off the heat. The carryover heat will wilt the spinach down.
4. Once the steak has rested a few minutes, thinly slice it. Serve over the top of the spinach mixture.

Nutritional Facts
Calories: 280 | Carbs: 11g | Fat: 13g | Protein: 28g

Fish & Seafood

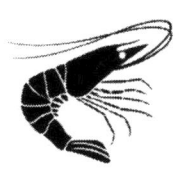

SHRIMP PICCATA W/ ZUCCHINI NOODLES

Servings: 4

Ingredients

- 2 tbsp. olive oil, extra virgin
- 2 garlic cloves, minced
- 1 lb. raw shrimp, peeled and de-veined
- 1 cup chicken broth, low sodium
- 1 tbsp. cornstarch
- ⅓ cup white wine
- ¼ cup lemon juice, fresh
- 3 tbsp. capers, drained and rinsed
- 2 tbsp. parsley, fresh, chopped

Directions

1. Cut the zucchini lengthwise and use your spiralizer or peeler to cut into noodles. Stop when you get to the seeds. Put noodles in colander and toss with salt. Let drain for 15 - 30 minutes. Then, squeeze out excess water.
2. Heat butter and 1 tbsp. oil in a skillet over medium heat. Add in the garlic and cook until fragrant. Then, add shrimp and cook, stirring for one minute.
3. Combine broth and cornstarch in a small bowl and whisk until combined. Add shrimp and then add the wine, lemon juice, and capers. Simmer, stirring occasionally until the shrimp is cooked all the way. Then, remove from heat.
4. Heat 1 tbsp. of the oil in a skillet over medium heat and add in the zucchini noodles. Toss until hot. Then, serve with shrimp and sauce over the noodles sprinkled with a little parsley.

Nutritional Facts
Calories: 280 | Carbs: 13g | Fat: 15g | Protein: 24g

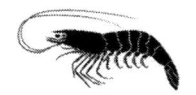

WALNUT CRUSTED SALMON

Servings: 4

Ingredients

- 2 tsp. Dijon mustard
- 1 garlic clove, minced
- ¼ tsp. lemon zest
- 1 tsp. rosemary, fresh, chopped
- ½ tsp. honey
- ½ tsp. salt
- ¼ tsp. red pepper flakes
- 3 tbsp. breadcrumbs, panko
- 3 tbsp. walnuts, finely chopped
- 1 tsp. olive oil, extra-virgin
- 1lb. salmon fillet, fresh or frozen

Directions

1. Preheat oven to 425°F. Line a baking sheet with parchment paper.
2. In a small bowl, combine the mustard, zest, juice, rosemary, honey, salt, and red pepper flakes. In another small bowl, combine panko, walnuts, and oil.
3. Set salmon onto the baking sheet and spread some of the mustard mixture on each piece. Once it's done, you can then top each fillet with the breadcrumb mix. Make sure to press it down gently until it sticks to the fish.
4. Bake until salmon is flaky (about 8 – 12 minutes).
5. Sprinkle with parsley and add a lemon wedge when you serve.

Nutritional Facts
Calories: 222 | Carbs: 4g | Fat: 12g | Protein: 24g

GREEK BAKED SHRIMP

Servings: 4

Ingredients

- 1 lb. large shrimp, peeled and de-veined
- ½ tsp. red pepper flakes
- ¼ tsp. kosher salt
- 3 tbsp. olive oil
- 1 med. onion, chopped
- 3 garlic cloves, minced
- 15 oz. canned crushed tomatoes
- ½ tsp. allspice, ground
- ½ tsp. cinnamon, ground
- ½ cup feta cheese, crumbled
- 2 tbsp. dill, fresh, chopped

Directions

1. Preheat oven to 375°F. Then, rinse and dry the shrimp. Place the shrimp in a bowl and season with salt, pepper, and pepper flakes.
2. Heat a heavy skillet with olive oil over medium heat. Then, add in garlic and onion and sauté until soft. Stir in the spice and cook until you smell the spices. Add in the tomatoes and let simmer for 20 minutes.
3. Take the skillet off the heat and place shrimp into the sauce. Crumble feta over the top. Then, bake for 15 - 18 minutes or until shrimp is fully cooked.
4. When done, sprinkle with dill. Serve with crusty bread.

Nutritional Facts
Calories: 241 | Carbs: 7.2g | Fat: 7.8g | Protein: 34.8g

BASS W/ TOMATOES AND OLIVES

Servings: 4

Ingredients

- 4 bass fillets
- Sea salt
- Herbs de Provence
- 1 tbsp. Dijon mustard
- 3 med. tomatoes, diced
- ⅓ cup olives, mixed, pitted, and chopped
- 1 tbsp. capers
- 1 garlic clove, minced
- 2 tbsp. olive oil
- 1 tbsp. white wine vinegar
- Parsley, chopped - garnish

Directions

1. Preheat the broiler.
2. Rinse fish and pat dry. Place the fish on the baking sheet. Season with salt and herbs de Provence. Spread a generous amount of Dijon mustard on top of each fillet.
3. Mix together the tomatoes, capers, garlic, olive oil, vinegar and ½ tsp. of salt in a medium bowl. Spoon the mixture over the fish.
4. Bake fish in the broiler for 10 minutes or until fish is cooked through. Rotate the pan or skillet halfway through.
5. Garnish with parsley.

Nutritional Facts
Calories: 577 | Carbs: 38g | Fat: 24g | Protein: 38g

COUSCOUS W/ TUNA

Servings: 4

Ingredients

- 1 cup chicken broth
- 1 ¼ cups couscous
- ¾ tsp. kosher salt
- 2 - 5 oz. cans oil-packed tuna
- 1-pint cherry tomatoes, halved
- ½ cup sliced pepperoncini
- ⅓ cup parsley, fresh, chopped
- ¼ cup capers
- Extra-virgin olive oil, for serving
- Kosher salt and pepper
- 1 lemon, quartered

Directions

1. Bring the broth to a boil in a small pot. Remove the pot from the heat, add in the couscous, and cover. Leave to stand for 10 minutes.
2. Combine the tuna, tomatoes, pepperoncini, parsley, and capers together in a medium bowl.
3. Uncover couscous and fluff it with a fork. Season with salt and pepper and drizzle with olive oil. Top the couscous with the tuna mixture and serve with lemon wedges.

Nutritional Facts
Calories: 226 | Carbs: 44g | Fat: 1g | Protein: 8g

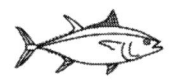

PARMESAN PESTO TILAPIA

Servings: 4

Ingredients

- 4 tilapia fillets
- ¼ cup basil pesto
- ½ cup parmesan cheese, freshly grated
- 1 cup tomatoes, chopped
- Salt, pepper, lemon juice, melted butter

Directions

1. Preheat the broiler. Pat the tilapia dry with a paper towel. Then, place each fillet onto a foil-lined baking sheet. Coat the fillet with oil before doing this to keep the fish from sticking.
2. Sprinkle each fillet with 2 tbsp. of parmesan cheese. Broil for 10-11 minutes or until the fish is cooked through.
3. Top each fillet with fresh tomatoes and pesto. You can also top with salt, pepper, lemon juice, and melted butter.

Nutritional Facts
Calories: 230 | Carbs: 4.6g | Fat: 11.2g | Protein: 27.9g

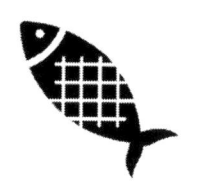

HONEY MUSTARD SALMON

Servings: 5

Ingredients

- 1 tbsp. raw honey
- 1 tbsp. coarse-grained mustard
- ½ tsp. white wine vinegar
- Sea salt and black pepper
- 1 - 2 lb. salmon fillet
- 2 ½ cups butternut squash, peeled, seeded, and cubed
- 12 oz. Brussel sprouts, trimmed and halved
- 2 cups cherry tomatoes
- 2 tbsp. avocado oil
- ½ tsp. lemon juice, fresh
- ¼ tsp. garlic powder
- ¼ tsp. onion powder
- ¾ tsp. oregano, dried
- ⅛ tsp. turmeric, ground
- 1 lemon, thinly sliced

Directions

1. Combine in a small bowl the honey, mustard, vinegar, ½ tsp. of oregano, ½ tsp. salt, and ¼ tsp. pepper and whisk until it is thoroughly mixed. Place the fillets in a baking dish and pour the marinade over the fish. Marinate for 15 minutes.
2. Preheat oven to 400°F. Then, in a large bowl combine squash, Brussel sprouts, tomatoes, oil, lemon juice, garlic powder, onion powder, the rest of the oregano, turmeric, salt, and pepper. Toss the vegetables until fully coated and then spread out on a baking sheet.
3. Remove the fish from the marinade and place it in the center of baking sheet. Keep excess marinade to baste while cooking. Roast the fish until it is flaky and the veggies are crispy, yet tender.

Nutritional Facts
Calories: 523 | Carbs: 23g | Fat: 31g | Protein: 41g

Vegetables

STUFFED PORTOBELLO MUSHROOMS CAPRESE STYLE

Servings: 4

Ingredients

- 1 garlic clove, minced
- ½ tsp. salt
- ½ tsp. pepper
- 4 portobello mushrooms, stems and gills removed
- 1 cup cherry tomatoes, halved
- ½ cup mozzarella pearls
- ½ cup basil, fresh, sliced
- 2 tsp. balsamic vinegar

Directions

1. Preheat the oven to 400°F. Then, combine 2 tbsp. of oil with garlic, ¼ tsp. salt, and ¼ tsp. pepper in a small bowl. Use a brush to coat the mushrooms. Next, place on a baking sheet and bake until soft.
2. In a medium bowl, combine the tomatoes, mozzarella, basil, salt, pepper, and oil. Fill the mushrooms with the mixture and bake for a further 12 minutes. Drizzle each mushroom with vinegar and serve.

Nutritional Facts
Calories: 186 | Carbs: 6g | Fat: 16g | Protein: 6g

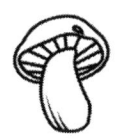

ZUCCHINI LASAGNA ROLLS

Servings: 6

Ingredients

- ¼ tsp. salt
- 2 cups crushed tomatoes
- 1 tsp. Italian seasoning
- 4 tsp. garlic, minced
- ¼ tsp. crushed red pepper flakes
- 2 ½ cups ricotta cheese, part-skim
- ¼ cup parmesan cheese, grated
- ½ tsp. pepper
- ¼ cup almonds, chopped

Directions

1. Preheat oven to 425°F. Spray two baking sheets with cooking spray.
2. Slice each zucchini lengthwise into 1/8" thick strips. Brush the strips with oil and sprinkle with salt. Place on one of the baking sheets and roast until soft. Then, reduce heat to 350°F.
3. Mix tomatoes, Italian seasoning, 2 tsp. garlic and crushed red peppers in a large bowl. Then, spread that mix into a baking dish.
4. Next, add the ricotta, parmesan, pepper, and garlic in another bowl. Once the zucchini is cool, spoon the ricotta into each slice and roll up and place seam down in the baking dish. Bake for 25-30 minutes.
5. While this is in the oven, put the almonds and the rest of the garlic, as well as some salt, into a food processor. Process until coarsely ground. Heat a bit of oil in a skillet and add the almond mix into it. Cook until it is fragrant and slightly browned. Serve as a topping.

Nutritional Facts
Calories: 324 | Carbs: 19g | Fat: 21g | Protein: 17g

STUFFED SWEET POTATOES

Servings: 4

Ingredients

- 4 lrg. sweet potatoes, washed and dried
- 2 tbsp. olive oil
- 1 sm. yellow onion, finely chopped
- ½ tsp kosher salt
- 15 oz. can black beans, drained and rinsed
- ¼ cup water
- 1 can chipotle in adobo chili, finely chopped
- 3 tsp. adobo sauce
- 1 med. lime, halved
- ½ cup Greek yogurt, whole-milk, plain

Directions

1. Line a baking sheet with aluminum foil. Stab the sweet potatoes with a fork in multiple spots. Spread on the baking sheet and bake until tender (about 1 hr.). Now, you can make the chipotle black beans.
2. Heat the oil in a skillet over medium heat. Then add in the onion and cook until soft and translucent. Sprinkle in salt.
3. Add the beans, water chipotle chile, and 1 tbsp. adobo sauce. Cover and let simmer for several minutes. Do this until the water has evaporated from the mixture. Remove from heat and take half a lime and squeeze into the mixture.
4. Now, mix yogurt with the remaining adobo sauce in a small bowl.
5. Once the potatoes are cooked, cut down the center and fill with black beans. Top with avocado, yogurt, and cilantro. Squeeze some lime juice over the top and serve.

> Nutritional Facts
> Calories: 427 | Carbs: 60.9g | Fat: 16.5g | Protein: 13.2g

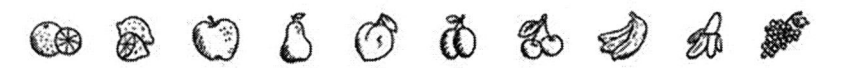

ROASTED STUFFED EGGPLANT

Servings: 4

Ingredients

- 2 sm. eggplants
- 2 tbsp. olive oil, extra-virgin
- 2 garlic cloves, chopped
- ¼ tsp. salt
- ½ tsp. ground pepper
- ½ cup parmesan cheese, finely grated
- 1 ¼ cup breadcrumbs
- 1 large egg, lightly beaten
- ⅓ cup parsley, fresh chopped
- 1 tsp. capers, rinsed
- 1 ¼ cups tomato sauce
- 4 lrg. basil leaves

Directions

1. Preheat the oven to 375 °F. Then, halve the eggplant lengthwise. Trim off a bit of underside to allow them to lay flat. Cut around the inside edge with a paring knife and separate the flesh from the skin. Scoop out the flesh and roughly chop. Set the shells aside.
2. In a medium saucepan over medium heat, warm 2 tbsp. of oil. Then, add in the meat of the eggplant and cook until soft. Add in the garlic and cook until fragrant. Move this to a bowl and season with salt and pepper. Let cool.
3. Heat ¼ cup of oil in the skillet. Season shells with salt, pepper, and 2 tbsp. of parmesan. Then, cook the shells until golden brown and soft. Drain on paper towels.
4. Dunk breadcrumbs in water and then squeeze them out. Place them in the bowl with the eggplant filling. Then add ¼ cup parmesan, egg, parsley, and capers. Mix well. Fill the eggplant shells with the stuffing.

5. Spread the tomato sauce on the bottom of a baking dish and then place the stuffed shells in the dish, as well. Spoon some of the sauce over the shells and top with a basil leaf. Sprinkle some parmesan on top. Bake until it is hot, about 25 minutes.

> *Nutritional Facts*
> *Calories: 324 | Carbs: 27g | Fat: 21g | Protein: 9g*

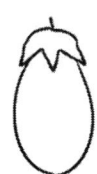

SLOW COOKER MINESTRONE

Servings: 6 - 8

Ingredients

- 4 med. carrots, peeled and sliced
- 2 celery stalks, sliced
- 1 lrg. onion, chopped
- ½ sm. head savoy cabbage, chopped
- 3 garlic cloves, minced
- 2- 15 oz. cans cannellini beans, drained, rinsed
- 14.5 oz. can dice tomatoes
- 6 cups water
- 1 pc. parmesan cheese rind (optional)
- 1 tbsp. kosher salt
- ½ tsp. pepper
- 1 sprig of rosemary, fresh
- 1 lrg. sprig of thyme, fresh
- 1 sprig of oregano, fresh
- 1 med. zucchini, chopped

Crouton Ingredients

- 8 oz. country bread, 1" cubes
- 3 tbsp. olive oil
- ½ tsp. kosher salt
- ½ tsp. black pepper
- 1 sprig of rosemary, fresh
- Parsley leaves, fresh chopped
- Red pepper flakes

Directions

1. Place all Ingredients except the zucchini in a large crockpot. Cover and cook on low for 6– 8 hours.
2. Remove the fresh herbs and the parmesan rind. Take 2 cups of soup out and place in blender. Puree herbs and rind and then return it to the soup and mix well. Add the zucchini and cook for a further 30 minutes.
3. Preheat oven to 400 ℉. Toss cubed bread in the olive oil, salt, and pepper in a large bowl. Spread out onto a baking sheet in a single layer. Scatter fresh herbs over the bread. Bake until the croutons are golden brown.

4. When the soup is done, use it to garnish as you serve.

> Nutritional Facts
> Calories: 292 | Carbs: 47.5g | Fat: 6.8g | Protein: 12.8g

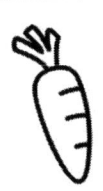

Salad

AVOCADO CAPRESE SALAD

Servings: 4

Ingredients

- 2 cups arugula, fresh
- 2-3 tomatoes, sliced
- ½ avocado, pitted and sliced
- 3 slices mozzarella cheese, fresh
- Basil leaves, fresh
- 1 tbsp. olive oil, extra-virgin
- 1 ½ tsp. balsamic vinegar
- Pinch of salt
- Dollop of honey
- Salt and pepper to taste

Directions

1. Combine together the arugula, tomato, avocado slices, and mozzarella in a serving bowl. Tear basil leaves and top the salad.
2. In a separate bowl, add in the olive oil, balsamic vinegar, sugar, honey, salt, pepper and whisk until emulsified. Coat salad to your taste and serve.

Nutritional Facts
Calories: 164 | Carbs: 11.6g | Fat: 11.8g | Protein: 5.4g

CHICKPEA AND HERB SALAD

Servings: 4

Ingredients

- 2 - 15 oz. cans chickpeas, rinsed, drained
- 1 med. red bell pepper, chopped
- 1 ½ cups parsley, fresh, chopped
- ½ cup celery plus leaves, chopped
- ½ cup red onion, chopped
- 3 tbsp. olive oil, extra-virgin
- 3 tbsp. fresh lemon juice
- 2 garlic cloves, minced
- ½ tsp. kosher salt and black pepper

Directions

1. In the serving bowl, add chickpeas, bell pepper, parsley, red onion, and celery.
2. Then, in a separate bowl, add olive oil, lemon juice, garlic, salt, pepper and whisk until emulsified. Dress salad and serve.

Nutritional Facts
Calories: 340 | Carbs: 44.4g | Fat: 13.7g | Protein: 12.1g

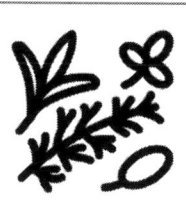

SUN-DRIED TOMATO AND FETA COUSCOUS SALAD

Servings: 4

Ingredients

- ⅓ cup pine nuts, shelled
- 1 tbsp. olive oil
- ½ tsp. kosher salt
- 1 ½ cup couscous
- ⅓ cup sun-dried tomatoes in oil, drained and diced
- ⅓ cup feta cheese, crumbled
- ¼ cup green onion, chopped

Directions

1. Heat the skillet over medium-high heat and toss in the pine nuts. Toast tossing frequently until golden brown.
2. In a medium saucepan, boil 1¼ cup water. Stir in couscous, olive oil, and salt. Remove from heat. Cover and let stand.
3. Using a fork, fluff the couscous and stir in the remaining Ingredients. Serve at room temperature.

Nutritional Facts
Calories: 327 | Carbs: 40g | Fat: 12g | Protein: 10g

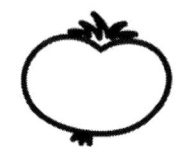

GREEK SALAD W/ AVOCADO

Servings: 8

Ingredients

- 2 cucumbers, peeled and cut ½" slices
- 1 ½ lbs. med. tomatoes, quartered
- ¼ sm. red onion, thinly sliced
- 1 ½ cups kalamata olives, pitted, halved
- ¼ cup parsley. Italian flat-leaf, chopped
- 2 avocados, pitted and cut into chunks
- 1 cup feta cheese, crumbled
- ½ cup olive oil, extra-virgin
- ½ cup red wine vinegar
- 2 garlic cloves, minced
- 1 tbsp. oregano
- 2 tsp. sugar
- 1 tsp. kosher salt
- 1 tsp. pepper

Directions

1. In a serving bowl, combine cucumbers, tomatoes, red onion, kalamata olives, and parsley. Place the avocados in a small bowl separate from the rest.
2. In a small bowl, combine the olive oil, red wine vinegar, garlic, oregano, sugar, salt, and pepper. Whisk until emulsified.
3. Take 1 tbsp. of dressing and coat the avocados. Pour the rest over the cucumber mixture and coat well. Add the avocado over the salad with feta cheese and serve.

Nutritional Facts
Calories: 440 | Carbs: 16g | Fat: 40g | Protein: 9g

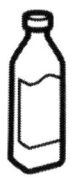

ARUGULA SALAD W/ PARMESAN

Servings: 2

Ingredients

- 2 tbsp. olive oil
- 2 tbsp. fresh lemon juice
- 1 tsp. honey
- ½ tsp. kosher salt
- ½ tsp. pepper
- 4 cups arugula
- ¼ cup parmesan cheese, shaved

Directions

1. In a serving bowl, combine the olive oil, lemon juice, honey, salt, and pepper. Whisk until emulsified. Add the arugula to the bowl and toss. Top with shaved parmesan and add pepper for taste.

Nutritional Facts
Calories: 164 | Carbs: 5.7g | Fat: 15.6g | Protein: 3.5g

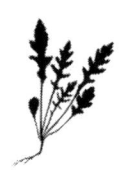

Snacks & Desserts

NO-BAKE MINT CHIP COOKIES

Servings: 12

Ingredients

- 2 cups coconut, shredded, unsweetened
- ½ cup coconut cream
- 2 tbsp. maple syrup
- 1 tsp. mint extract
- ½ tsp. spirulina
- ¼ cup cocoa nibs
- 1 cup chocolate chips

Directions

1. In the food processor, add in coconut and process until finely ground. Then, add in the coconut cream, sweetener, mint extract, and spirulina. Process until it all comes together in a sticky dough.
2. Add the cocoa nibs and blend briefly to mix them.
3. Scoop with ice cream scoop and shape into cookies. Place in the freezer for 15 minutes until hard. Melt chocolate chips in glass mixing bowl over simmering water. Then, dip frozen cookie in the chocolate. Sprinkle with more cocoa nibs and freeze again until firm.

Nutritional Facts
Calories: 209 | Carbs: 17g | Fat: 18g | Protein: 2g

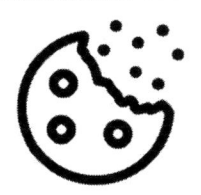

GRAIN-FREE HUMMINGBIRD CAKE

Servings: 16

Ingredients

- 2 med. bananas, overripe and smashed
- ¼ cup avocado oil
- ½ cup honey
- 4 eggs
- ¾ cup crushed pineapple
- 2 tsp. vanilla extract
- 3 cups almond flour
- ½ tsp. salt
- 2 tsp. baking soda
- 4 cups coconut whipped cream

Directions

1. Preheat oven to 350 ℉. Grease two 8" cake pans and set to the side.
2. Combine all Ingredients into a large bowl and mix until thoroughly combined.
3. Divide batter into each cake pan and smooth the top of the batter.
4. Bake for 30 – 35 minutes until the top starts to darken and the center is set.
5. Remove from the oven and let cool. Then, frost with your favorite frosting. Store in refrigerator.

Nutritional Facts
Calories: 347 | Carbs: 32g | Fat: 23g | Protein: 7g

PUMPKIN CHIA SEED PUDDING

Servings: 4

Ingredients

- 1 ¼ cup milk
- 1 cup pumpkin puree
- ½ cup chia seeds
- ¼ cup maple syrup
- 2 tsp. pumpkin spice
- ¼ cup sunflower seeds
- ¼ cup almonds, sliced
- ¼ cup blueberries, fresh

Directions

1. Add all the Ingredients in a bowl and thoroughly mix. Spoon into canning jars and refrigerate overnight.
2. Then, serve with either almonds, sunflower seeds, or blueberries.

> Nutritional Facts
> Calories: 189 | Carbs: 27g | Fat: 7.6g | Protein: 5.9g

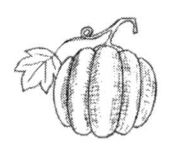

BAKED ZUCCHINI CHIPS

Servings: 8

Ingredients

- 4 zucchini squash, sliced 1/8" rounds
- Kosher salt
- Olive oil, extra-virgin
- Harissa spices

Directions

1. Thinly slice the zucchini with a mandolin. Lay out on some paper towels and sprinkle with salt. Then, cover with more paper towels and place a cutting board on top. Let stand for 15 – 20 minutes.
2. Preheat oven to 245°F. Line the sheet pan with parchment paper and lightly oil with olive oil. Then, lay the zucchini chips out onto the parchment paper in a single layer.
3. Brush each chip with olive oil and sprinkle with harissa. Bake in the oven for about 2 hours until crisp and golden. Serve with tzatziki at room temperature.

Nutritional Facts
Calories: 26 | Carbs: 1.9g | Fat: 1.9g | Protein: .8g

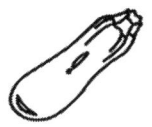

SUN-DRIED TOMATO AND GOAT CHEESE SPREAD

Servings: 1 cup

Ingredients

- ⅓ cup sun-dried tomatoes, oil-packed
- 2 garlic cloves, halved
- 1 tbsp. basil, fresh, minced
- 1 tbsp. parsley, fresh, minced
- 8 oz. goat cheese, cubed

Directions

1. Drain the sun-dried tomatoes, reserving 2 tsp. of the oil. Combine the garlic, basil, and parsley. Process until combined.
2. Then, add goat cheese, the sun-dried tomatoes, and oil. Cover and run through process until smooth. Chill until ready to serve. Serve with pita chips or fresh vegetables.

Nutritional Facts
Calories: 55 | Carbs: 2g | Fat: 4g | Protein: 3g

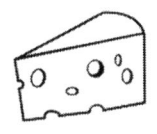

30 DAYS LOSE WEIGHT CHALLENGE

DAY 1

Breakfast: Eggs w/ Ratatouille

Servings: 2

Ingredients

- 1 tbsp. olive oil
- 1 sm. onion, thinly slice and halved
- 1 garlic clove, minced
- 2 med. zucchini
- 2 med. tomatoes, chopped
- ½ tsp. thyme, fresh
- 1 tsp. paprika
- 1 med. red bell pepper
- Salt and pepper
- 2 lrg. eggs

Directions

1. In a large skillet, heat oil on medium heat. Then, add the onion and cook until softened. Add the garlic and cook until fragrant. Once that is done, add the squash and cook until soft and brown. Next, you will add the tomatoes, thyme, and paprika. Then, let simmer until it thickens, about 20 minutes.

2. While you are doing this, roast the red pepper on the stovetop. Once you have done that, let it cool and remove the core and seeds. Remove skillet from heat and add pepper. Then, salt and pepper to taste. Let the dish cool while frying the eggs. Serve with the egg on top.

> *Nutritional Facts*
> Calories: 226 | Carbs: 20.6g | Fat: 12.5g | Protein: 11.1g

Lunch: Greek Turkey Burger (see page 242)

Dinner: Grilled Balsamic Chicken w/ Olive Tapenade (see page 238)

DAY 2

Breakfast: Avocado Toast Caprese Style (see page 229)

Lunch: Cauliflower Salad w/ Dressing

Servings: 4

Ingredients

- 1 med. head cauliflower
- 1 tsp. olive oil
- ½ tsp. kosher salt
- ¼ cup shallot, chopped fine
- 3 tbsp. fresh lemon juice
- 2 tbsp. tahini
- ½ cup parsley, flat-leaf, chopped
- ¼ cup dried cherries, chopped
- 1 tbsp. Mint, fresh, chopped
- 3 tbsp. pistachios, roasted, salted, chopped

Directions

1. Grate cauliflower into a large microwaveable bowl. Add in olive oil and ¼ tsp. of salt. Cover with plastic wrap and microwave for 3 minutes. Spread cauliflower over a baking sheet and leave to cool.
2. In a large mixing bowl, add the chopped shallot and lemon juice. Let sit for several minutes. Then, stir in the tahini. Pour cauliflower into the mixture and toss. Add in parsley, mint, cherries, and ¼ tsp. of salt and combine.
3. Serve sprinkled with chopped pistachios.

Nutritional Facts
Calories: 165 | Carbs: 20g | Fat: 8g | Protein: 6g

Dinner: Pork Scaloppini w/ Lemon and Capers (see page 240)

DAY 3

Breakfast: Frittata w/ Asparagus, Mushroom, & Goat Cheese (see page 230)

Lunch: Skewered Beef w/ Garlicky White Bean Sauce (see page 246)

Dinner: Chicken Skillet w/ Bulgur

Servings: 4

Ingredients

- 4 chicken breasts, boneless, skinless
- ¾ tsp. kosher salt
- ½ tsp. pepper
- 1 tbsp. olive oil
- 1 cup red onion, thinly sliced
- 1 tbsp. garlic, sliced thin
- ½ cup uncooked bulgur
- 2 tsp. oregano, dried, chopped
- 4 cups kale, fresh, chopped
- ½ cup roasted red peppers, jarred, sliced
- 1 cup chicken stock, unsalted
- 2 oz. feta, crumbled
- 1 tbsp. dill fresh, chopped

Directions

1. Preheat oven to 400°F. Season chicken breasts with salt and pepper. Heat 1 ½ tsp. of oil in a skillet over medium-high heat. Add chicken to the heated pan and cook until browned on both sides. Remove chicken.
2. Add leftover oil, onion, and garlic to skillet. Cook until soft and garlic is fragrant. Add bulgur and oregano. Cook until the bulgur is toasted. Add in kale and pepper and cook until kale is wilted. Add stock and ¼ tsp. of both salt and pepper. Bring to a boil and remove from heat.
3. Place chicken back in skillet, put in the oven and bake until the chicken juices run clear. Remove from oven, sprinkle feta and dill over the top, then serve.

Nutritional Facts
Calories: 369 | Carbs: 21g | Fat: 11.3g | Protein: 45g

DAY 4

Breakfast: Spinach Feta Breakfast Wrap

Servings: 4

Ingredients

- 10 lrg. eggs
- ½ lb. baby spinach
- 4 whole-wheat tortillas
- ½ pint grape tomatoes, halved
- 4 oz. feta cheese, crumbled
- Butter or olive oil
- Salt
- Pepper

Directions

1. In a large bowl, combine eggs and whisk until fully incorporated. Heat a large skillet over medium-high heat and add in either butter or olive oil to coat the bottom. When it is hot/melted, pour in the eggs and stir periodically until cooked. Add a pinch of salt and a healthy amount of pepper. Then, remove from pan and set aside.
2. Clean skillet out and then return to medium-high heat, add more oil/butter. Add in the spinach and cook until wilted down. Remove from skillet and allow to cool.
3. Place tortilla on cutting board and add about ¼ of the eggs, spinach, tomatoes, and feta in the middle. Wrap the burrito tight and serve. (You can wrap them in aluminum foil and store them in your freezer in freezer bags, as well.)

Nutritional Facts
Calories: 543 | Carbs: 46.5g | Fat: 27.0g | Protein: 28.1g

Lunch: Couscous w/ Tuna (see page 262)

Dinner: Pomegranate Citrus Glazed Duck Breast (see page 244)

DAY 5

Breakfast: Poached Egg with Greens & White Beans (see page 232)

Lunch: Shrimp Pasta (see page 123)

Servings: 8

Ingredients

- 12 oz. pasta, bow tie
- 1 ½ lbs. shrimp, fresh, peeled, deveined
- ¼ cup butter
- 3 garlic cloves, minced
- 12 oz. jar roasted red peppers, drained, chopped
- 1 cup artichoke hearts, quartered
- ½ cup white wine, dry
- 3 tbsp. capers, drained
- ½ cup whipping cream
- 1 tsp. lemon zest
- 2 tbsp. lemon juice
- ¾ cup feta, crumbled
- 2 oz. pine nuts, toasted
- ¼ cup basil, fresh, torn

Directions

1. In the Dutch oven, cook pasta according to instructions. Then, drain and return to Dutch oven and cover to keep warm.
2. Heat butter in a skillet over medium-high heat and then add garlic. Cook until fragrant, then add shrimp. Cook for 2 minutes, then add in red peppers, artichokes, wine, and capers.
3. Bring this to a boil, then turn down the heat and let simmer uncovered until the shrimp is cooked thoroughly. Stir in cream, lemon zest, and juice. Let return to boil. Reduce heat and let simmer for another minute.
4. Combine shrimp mixture with pasta and toss gently.
5. Serve sprinkled with feta, pine nuts, and basil.

> *Nutritional Facts*
> *Calories: 322 | Carbs: 28.5g | Fat: 18.5g | Protein: 12.7g*

Dinner: Chicken w/ Tomato and Balsamic Sauce (see page 250)

DAY 6

Breakfast: Start Your Morning Right Grain Salad (see page 234)

Lunch: Stuffed Sweet Potatoes (see page 268)

Dinner: Caprese Chicken

Servings: 2

Ingredients

- 2 chicken breasts, boneless, skinless
- Kosher salt and pepper for taste
- 1 tbsp. olive oil, extra-virgin
- 1 tbsp. butter
- 1 jar basil pesto of your choice
- 4 oz. mozzarella, grated
- 1 cup grape tomatoes, halved
- ½ cup balsamic glaze
- ⅓ cup basil, fresh, chopped

Directions

1. Preheat oven to 400 ℉. Slice chicken in half lengthwise and season with salt and pepper on both sides of each breast. Heat skillet with oil and butter over medium-high heat. Then, add the chicken breasts and cook on both sides until lightly browned.
2. Spoon pesto over the top of each chicken breast and top with grated mozzarella, as well as some tomatoes. Place skillet in oven and let bake for 10-12 minutes until chicken is done. Remove and garnish with basil and balsamic glaze.

Nutritional Facts
Calories: 199 | Carbs: 7.3g | Fat: 16.6g | Protein: 6.8g

DAY 7

Breakfast: Breakfast Pizza

Servings: 4

Ingredients

- 1 lrg. avocado
- 1 tbsp. cilantro, fresh, chopped
- 1 ½ tsp. fresh lime juice
- ⅛ tsp. salt
- ½ lb. pizza dough, pre-made
- 4 lrg. eggs
- 1 tbsp. olive oil
- Hot sauce, for serving

Directions

1. Cut the avocado and scoop out the flesh into medium bowl. Add in cilantro, lime juice, and salt. Mash until your desired consistency. Taste and add seasonings to your preference.
2. Split dough into 4 parts. Flour cutting board and roll each piece into about a 6" pie.
3. Heat a cast-iron skillet over medium-high heat and then place one pizza crust in the skillet. Cook until the dough is browned, and the surface begins to bubble. Flip and repeat on the other side. Use a spatula to press down if it puffs up. Remove and set aside. Repeat with the other pieces of dough.
4. Spread avocado mixture evenly over pizza dough.
5. Heat a small frying pan over medium heat. Fry eggs to your preference and then top pizza with them. Serve hot with/without a drizzle of hot sauce.

Nutritional Facts
Calories: 337 | Carbs: 33.2g | Fat: 17.6g | Protein: 12.3g

Lunch: Chickpea & Herb Salad (see page 275)

Dinner: Mediterranean Spaghetti Squash w/ Turkey (see page 252)

DAY 8

Breakfast: Easy Muesli (see page 236)

Lunch: Falafel and Tomato Salad

Servings: 4

Ingredients

- ¼ cup olive oil, extra-virgin
- 2 tbsp. red wine vinegar
- ½ tsp. kosher salt
- ½ tsp. pepper
- 2 lbs. tomatoes, sliced ½"
- 4 cups arugula
- 1 cup cucumber, sliced
- ¾ cup red onion, thinly sliced
- ½ cup mint, fresh, torn
- 4 cooked falafel patties
- 2 oz. feta, crumbled
- ¼ cup pine nuts, toasted

Directions

1. Combine the oil, vinegar, salt, and pepper in a large bowl. Whisk until emulsified. Add in tomatoes and toss to coat. Let it stand for a few minutes. Place tomatoes on the serving plate. Reserve rest of vinaigrette.
2. Add arugula, cucumber, onion, mint, and falafel to the vinaigrette in the bowl. Toss gently. Arrange the falafel mixture over the tomatoes. Sprinkle feta and toasted pine nuts. Drizzle any remaining vinaigrette over the top.

Nutritional Facts
Calories: 386 | Carbs: 32g | Fat: 25.1g | Protein: 12g

Dinner: Boneless Pork Chops w/ Vegetables (see page 254)

DAY 9

Breakfast: Eggs w/ Ratatouille (see page 286)
Lunch: Arugula Salad w/ Parmesan (see page 278)
Dinner: Grilled Eggplant Skillet

Servings: 4

Ingredients

- 7 tbsp. olive oil
- 14 oz. packaged tofu, extra firm, cubed
- 1 lrg. eggplant, sliced ½" thick
- 28 oz. can tomatoes, whole, peeled, drained and chopped
- 2 garlic cloves, grated
- 1 tsp. oregano, fresh, chopped
- ½ tsp. cinnamon, ground
- ½ tsp. cumin, ground
- ¼ tsp. kosher salt
- ¼ tsp. red pepper flakes
- 3 tbsp. feta, crumbled
- ⅓ cup mint, fresh, chopped

Directions

1. Preheat broiler.
2. In a large oven-safe skillet, heat 2 tbsp. of oil over medium-high heat. Add tofu and cook until browned. Remove tofu and add ¼ cup of oil. Lay eggplant slices in the skillet and cook until brown. Flip and repeat the process. Remove skillet from heat.
3. Combine tomatoes, garlic, seasoning in a medium bowl. Top the eggplant with the tofu and spoon mixture over the top of that. Drizzle top with olive oil and sprinkle feta.
4. Place skillet in oven and broil for about 4 minutes. Remove garnish with mint and oregano, then serve.

Nutritional Facts
Calories: 397 | Carbs: 20g | Fat: 31g | Protein: 14g

DAY 10

Breakfast: Frittata w/ Spinach and Artichoke

Servings: 4 - 6

Ingredients

- 10 lrg. eggs
- ½ cup sour cream, full fat
- 1 tbsp. Dijon mustard
- 1 tsp. kosher salt
- ¼ tsp. black pepper
- 1 cup parmesan cheese, grated
- 2 tbsp. olive oil
- 14 oz. can artichoke hearts, drained, dried, and quartered
- 5 oz. baby spinach, fresh
- 2 garlic cloves, minced

Directions

1. Preheat oven to 400°F. In a large bowl, combine together the eggs, sour cream, mustard, salt, pepper, and ½ cup parmesan cheese. Whisk until combined thoroughly.
2. Heat the skillet over medium heat with oil until oil is hot. Then, add in the artichokes and cook until lightly browned. Next, add in spinach and garlic. Toss until spinach is wilted and the liquid is gone.
3. Spread the mix evenly in one layer across the bottom of the skillet and then add the egg mixture. Sprinkle rest of parmesan over the top. Tilt skillet to make sure the mix is evenly distributed over the vegetables. Cook until the edges of the eggs begin to brown and pull from edge of skillet.
4. Then, remove from stove and put in the oven. Bake for 12 - 15 minutes more until done. Let cool for a few minutes, then slice and serve.

Nutritional Facts
Calories: 316 | Carbs: 6.4g | Fat: 25.9g | Protein: 17.9g

Lunch: Cauliflower Salad w/ Dressing (see page 125)

Dinner: Walnut Crusted Salmon (see page 259)

DAY 11

Breakfast: Spinach Feta Breakfast Wrap (see page)

Lunch: Chicken Quinoa Bowl

Servings: 2

Ingredients

- 1 chicken breast, boneless, skinless, cubed
- ¼ cup olive oil + 2 tbsp.
- 1 lemon, juiced and zested
- 2 garlic cloves, minced
- 2 tsp. oregano, dried
- 1 ½ tsp. kosher salt
- ¼ tsp pepper
- 1 cup broccoli, roasted
- ½ cup tomatoes, roasted
- 1 cup quinoa, dried
- 1 cup feta, crumbled

Directions

1. Preheat oven to 400 °F. Coat tomatoes and broccoli with oil, salt, and pepper and spread out over baking sheets. Roast until soft and lightly browned. Take out and let cool.
2. Slice chicken breast into 1" chunks and place in a freezer bag. Combine olive oil, lemon juice and zest, garlic, oregano, salt, pepper and whisk until fully combined. Add to freezer bag and let marinate for at least 30 minutes.
3. In a skillet, heat 2 tbsp. of oil over medium-high heat. Add the chicken and cook until brown on all sides. Reduce heat and add the broccoli and tomatoes with more olive oil if need be. Warm all the way through.
4. Rinse your quinoa while bringing a pan of water to a boil. Add in 1 tsp. of salt and the quinoa. Boil until al dente. Then, drain and fluff. Return to pan and let sit for 5-10 minutes.
5. Assemble bowls and sprinkle with feta, then serve.

Nutritional Facts
Calories: 810 | Carbs: 69.4g | Fat: 50g | Protein: 27.2g

Dinner: Greek Baked Shrimp (see page 260)

DAY 12

Breakfast: Breakfast Pizza (see page 197)

Lunch: Shrimp Pasta (see page 123)

Dinner: Crock Pot Cacciatore

Servings: 10

Ingredients

- 10 chicken thighs, skinless, bone-in
- Kosher salt and pepper to taste
- Olive oil, extra virgin
- 5 garlic cloves, chopped fine
- ½ lrg. onion, chopped
- 28 oz. can crushed tomatoes
- ½ med. bell pepper, green, chopped
- ½ med. bell pepper, red, chopped
- 8 oz. mushrooms, sliced
- 2 sprigs of thyme, fresh
- 2 bay leaves
- ⅓ cup parsley, fresh, chopped
- ½ cup parmesan, grated

Directions

1. Season the chicken with salt and pepper liberally. Heat the olive oil in a skillet over a medium-high heat. Add in the seasoned chicken and cook until nicely browned on both sides. Add into the crockpot.
2. Return skillet to heat and add in a little more oil. Then, toss in the garlic and onion and cook until soft. Add this to the crockpot. Do the same for bell peppers and tomatoes.

3. Cover and cook in crockpot on low for 8 hours. Remove bay leaves and remove the chicken from the sauce. Pull the meat from the bones and put the meat back into the crockpot, stirring it thoroughly. Add in the parsley. Serve over pasta with parmesan sprinkled on top.

> Nutritional Facts
> Calories: 90 | Carbs: 7g | Fat: 4g | Protein: 7g

DAY 13

Breakfast: Smoked Salmon & Poached Eggs on Toast

Servings: 2

Ingredients

- 2 slices of multigrain bread
- ½ lrg. avocado
- ¼ tsp. fresh lemon juice
- Pinch of salt and pepper
- 3 ½ oz. salmon, smoked
- 2 eggs
- 2 slices of tomato
- ¼ cup microgreens

Directions

1. Poach eggs. Simmer water in a saucepan with a splash of vinegar. Stir it to create a whirlpool and then drop the egg into the water. Cook for 2-3 minutes and then move carefully with ladle to paper towel. Let stand there while you do the rest.
2. Cut and scoop out the flesh of half of an avocado into a small bowl. Mash with lemon juice, salt, and pepper.
3. Toast the bread. Then, spread avocado mixture evenly. Add the smoked salmon and poached egg.
4. Place the tomato and microgreens on the toast and serve.

Nutritional Facts
Calories: 471 | Carbs: 41.3g | Fat: 22g | Protein: 27.4g

Lunch: Falafel & Tomato Salad (see page 276)

Dinner: Stuffed Portobello Mushroom Caprese Style (see page 266)

DAY 14

Breakfast: Avocado Toast Caprese Style (see page 229)

Lunch: Tuna Melt w/ Olive Salsa

Servings: 4

Ingredients

- ⅓ cup green olives, pitted
- 1 tbsp. olive oil, extra-virgin
- 2 tsp. lemon zest
- 3 tbsp. fresh lemon juice
- 2 tbsp. parsley, fresh, chopped
- 1 tbsp. sunflower seeds, toasted
- ¼ tsp. kosher salt
- ¼ tsp. pepper
- ¼ tsp. red pepper flakes
- 5 oz. can tuna, in water, drained
- 2 tbsp. dill, fresh, chopped
- 2 tbsp. Greek yogurt, plain, whole milk
- 1 tsp. Dijon mustard
- 1 ½ oz. mozzarella, grated
- 4 slices whole-grain bread

Directions

1. Combine olives, 1 tsp. lemon zest, 1 tbsp. lemon juice, parsley sunflower seed, and pepper flakes and stir well.
2. Mix tuna, dill, mayonnaise, mustard, 1 tsp. zest, 1 tbsp. juice, salt, and pepper until well combined.
3. Preheat broiler. Lay out bread and top with tuna mixture. Sprinkle on cheese and broil for 2 minutes. Remove top with olive salsa and serve.

Nutritional Facts
Calories: 221 | Carbs: 14g | Fat: 11g | Protein: 16g

Dinner: Zucchini Lasagna Rolls (see page 267)

DAY 15

Breakfast: Frittata w/ Asparagus, Mushroom & Goat Cheese (see page 230)

Lunch: Chicken Quinoa Bowl (see page 297)

Dinner: Roasted Salmon w/ Vegetables and Citrus

Servings: 4

Ingredients

- 1 ½ lb. salmon fillet
- 2 blood oranges, wedged
- 1 navel orange, wedged
- 1 sm. red onion, wedged
- 1 med. golden beet, sliced 1/8"
- 1 sm. red beet, sliced 1/8"
- 1 lrg. carrot, sliced 1/8"
- 2 tbsp. olive oil
- 1 tsp. fennel seeds, crushed
- ½ tsp. kosher salt
- 2 tbsp. fresh lemon juice
- 2 tsp. tarragon, fresh, chopped

Directions

1. Preheat oven to 450°F. Dry fish and place on a parchment-lined baking sheet. Arrange oranges and vegetables around it. Combine the oil, fennel seeds, salt, and pepper in a bowl. Drizzle oil over fish and vegetables.
2. Bake for 10-12 minutes until the fish flakes. Sprinkle lemon juice and tarragon over top and serve.

Nutritional Facts
Calories: 390 | Carbs: 21g | Fat: 17g | Protein: 38g

DAY 16

Breakfast: Ricotta Spread w/ Fruit

Servings: 4-6

Ingredients

- 1 cup ricotta, whole milk
- ½ cup almonds, sliced
- ¼ tsp. almond extract
- 1 tsp. honey
- Zest from orange

For serving

- 2 pieces of bread
- Sliced peaches (or any fruit)
- almonds

Directions

1. Mix ricotta, almonds, and almond extract in a bowl until combined completely. Add extra almonds and drizzle honey over the top.
2. Spread 1 spoon of mixture on each slice of bread and add peaches, almonds, and honey.

Nutritional Facts
Calories: 64 | Carbs: 3.5g | Fat: 8.3g | Protein: 7.1g

Lunch: Chicken Kebabs (see page 248)

Dinner: Shrimp Piccata w/ Zucchini Noodles (see page 258)

DAY 17

Breakfast: Start Your Morning Right Grain Salad (see page 234)

Lunch: Hearts of Palm and Tomato Salad

Servings: 4

Ingredients

- 3 cups cherry tomatoes, halved
- 15 oz. can hearts of palm, drained, sliced
- ¼ cup red onion, sliced thin
- ¼ cup parsley, chopped
- ¼ cup olive oil
- 1 ½ tbsp. red wine vinegar
- 1 tsp. sugar
- 1 tsp. kosher salt
- ½ tsp. pepper

Directions

1. Combine all vegetables and fresh herbs together.
2. In a separate bowl, combine the oil, vinegar, sugar, salt, and pepper and whisk until emulsified. Toss into vegetable mixture and serve.

Nutritional Facts
Calories: 133 | Carbs: 2.8g | Fat: 13.7g | Protein: .3g

Dinner: Roasted Stuffed Eggplant (see page 269)

DAY 18

Breakfast: Easy Muesli (see page 236)

Lunch: Garlic Steak w/ Warm Spinach (see page 256)

Dinner: Olive, Caper, and Lemon Chicken

Servings: 6

Ingredients

- 2 lemons, sliced ¼"
- ¼ cup olive oil, extra-virgin
- 6 chicken thighs, boneless
- 2 tbsp. flour, all-purpose
- 1 garlic clove, minced
- 1 cup chicken broth
- ¾ cup green olives
- ¼ cup capers
- 2 tbsp. butter
- 2 tbsp. parsley
- Kosher salt and pepper to taste

Directions

1. In a large skillet, heat 1 tbsp. of oil. Add in lemon slices and sear until browned. Remove and let sit. Season chicken and dredge in flour. Shake off excess. Add 1 ½ tbsp. of oil into the skillet and then place chicken thighs in skillet. Cook until golden brown on both sides. Remove from skillet and leave to rest with the lemon slices.

2. Add in more olive oil and garlic. Cook until fragrant. Add in the broth capers and olives, as well as the chicken and lemons. Let simmer until broth reduces by half. Then, add butter and parsley. Cook for another minute and then season with salt and pepper. Remove from heat and serve.

> *Nutritional Facts*
> *Calories: 147 | Carbs: 3.9g | Fat: 10.6g | Protein: 9.2g*

DAY 19

Breakfast: Baked Eggs w/ Avocado and Feta

Servings: 2

Ingredients

- 4 eggs
- 1 lrg. avocado
- Olive oil
- 3 tbsp. feta, crumbled
- Salt and pepper for taste

Directions

1. Break eggs into a ramekin and let come to room temperature.
2. Preheat oven to 400°F and place gratin dishes on the baking sheet. Heat them in oven for 10 minutes.
3. Cut avocado and slice. Remove dishes from oven and coat with olive oil. Place slices of avocado on the bottom of the dish and carefully pour two eggs in each.
4. Sprinkle feta, salt and pepper over the top.
5. Bake for 12-15 minutes and serve.

Nutritional Facts
Calories: 282 | Carbs: 14.4g | Fat: 38.1g | Protein: 23.5g

Lunch: Slow Cooker Minestrone (see page 271)

Dinner: Pork Scaloppini w/ Lemon and Capers (see page 240)

DAY 20

Breakfast: Ricotta Spread w/ Fruit (see page 303)
Lunch: Lentil Patties w/ Mint Yogurt Sauce

Servings: 4

Ingredients

- 2 ½ tbsp. olive oil
- ½ cup onion, chopped
- 1 tbsp. garlic, minced
- ¾ cup rolled oats
- 2 tbsp. red wine vinegar
- 1 tsp. kosher salt
- ½ tsp pepper
- 2 lrg. eggs
- 1 pkg. brown lentils, steamed
- 2 cups arugula
- 2 cups baby spinach
- ¾ cup yogurt, Greek, plain
- 2 tbsp. fresh lemon juice
- 2 tbsp. mint, fresh, chopped
- 3 tbsp. pistachios, unsalted, chopped

Directions

1. Heat 1 ½ tsp. oil over medium heat in a large skillet. Add onion and garlic and cook until soft and fragrant. Combine this mixture with oats, 1 tbsp. vinegar, ¾ tsp. salt, pepper, eggs, and lentils into a food processor. Pulse until combined. Make into patties and let sit for a few minutes.
2. Add 1 ½ tsp. of oil into skillet and cook patties in batches until both sides of each pattie are golden brown.
3. Mix 1 tbsp. vinegar and 1 tbsp. oil and whisk together. Toss with spinach and arugula until coated.
4. In a bowl, add together ½ tsp. salt, yogurt, juice, and mint.

5. Lay a bed of greens and add the lentil cakes. Serve with chopped pistachios and yogurt sauce.

Nutritional Facts
Calories: 413 | Carbs: 43g | Fat: 18g | Protein: 23g

Dinner: Bass w/ Tomatoes & Olives (see page 261)

DAY 21

Breakfast: Smoked Salmon & Poached Eggs on Toast (see page 300)

Lunch: Avocado Caprese Salad (see page 274)

Dinner: Pounded Chicken with Almond Paprika Vinaigrette

Servings: 4

Ingredients

- 4 chicken breasts, boneless, skinless
- ⅜ tsp. kosher salt
- ¼ tsp. pepper
- 3 tbsp. olive oil
- ¼ cup chicken stock, unsalted
- 1 garlic clove, minced
- 2 tbsp. water
- ¼ tsp. lemon zest
- 1 tbsp. lemon juice
- ¼ tsp. paprika, smoked
- ¼ tsp. Dijon mustard
- 2 tbsp. parsley, chopped
- 1 oz. green olives, chopped
- 2 tbsp. almonds, unsalted, roasted, chopped

Directions

1. Place chicken breast between a sheet of plastic wrap and pound until ¼" thick with meat mallet. Season both sides of the breast with salt and pepper.
2. Heat 1 ½ tsp. oil in a large skillet over medium-high heat. Add in chicken breasts and cook until brown on both sides. Remove when done and set aside.
3. In the same skillet, add stock and reduce heat. Scrape up the browned bits and stir in 2 tbsp. of oil. Also, add in garlic and cook until fragrant. Then, add in ⅛ tsp. of salt, almonds, water, lemon juice, paprika, and mustard. Cook for a few minutes. Spoon the sauce over the chicken, sprinkle parsley and olives over the top, and serve.

Nutritional Facts
Calories: 160 | Carbs: 4.4g | Fat: 15.8g | Protein: 2.1g

DAY 22

Breakfast: Pancakes w/ Greek Yogurt

Servings: 6

Ingredients

- 1 ¼ cup flour, all-purpose
- ¼ tsp. salt
- 2 tsp. baking powder
- 1 tsp. baking soda
- ¼ cup of sugar
- 3 tbsp. butter, unsalted, melted
- 3 eggs
- 1 ½ cups Greek yogurt, plain, non-fat
- ½ cup milk
- ½ cup blueberries (or other fruit)

Directions

1. Add flour, salt, baking powder, and baking soda to a large bowl and whisk until incorporated. In a separate bowl, add the sugar, melted butter, eggs, Greek yogurt, and milk. Whisk this mixture until combined fully. Slowly add the wet Ingredients to dry until fully combined. Let stand for 20 minutes.
2. Heat the griddle and spray with no-stick spray. Use a ¼ cup measuring cup to pour batter onto the griddle. Cook until bubbles appear and then flip. Once fully browned on both sides, remove pancakes. Repeat the process until all the batter is gone.
3. Top with more yogurt and fruit, then serve.

Nutritional Facts
Calories: 258 | Carbs: 33g | Fat: 8g | Protein: 11g

Lunch: Grilled Eggplant Skillet (see page 295))

Dinner: Chicken Skillet w/ Bulgur (see page 288)

DAY 23

Breakfast: Frittata w/ Spinach and Artichoke (see page 296)

Lunch: Crock Pot Kale and Turkey Meatball Soup

Servings: 10

Ingredients

- ¼ cup milk
- 2 slices bread
- 1 lb. turkey, ground
- 1 med. shallot, chopped fine
- ½ tsp. nutmeg, fresh grated
- 1 tsp. oregano
- ¼ tsp. red pepper flakes
- Kosher salt and pepper to taste
- ½ cup parmesan, grated
- 2 tbsp. parsley, chopped
- 1 egg, beaten
- 1 tbsp. olive oil
- 8 cups chicken broth
- 15 oz. white beans, drained, rinsed
- 2 carrots, sliced
- ½ onion, chopped
- 4 cups kale

Directions

1. Add milk into the mixing bowl. Rip bread apart and soak in milk. Then add turkey, shallot, nutmeg, oregano, pepper flakes, salt, pepper, cheese, parsley, and egg. Mix well until combined. Use a scoop to form 1/2" meatballs.
2. Heat the oil in a large skillet over medium-high heat. Then, sear meatballs in batches.
3. Add broth, beans, and the vegetables into crockpot. Drop meatballs in and cook on low for 4 hours.
4. Serve with red pepper flakes, parsley, and parmesan cheese sprinkled on top.

Nutritional Facts
Calories: 446 | Carbs: 6.4g | Fat: 21.7g | Protein: 53.4g

Dinner: Greek Turkey Burgers (see page 242)

DAY 24

Breakfast: Baked Eggs w/ Avocado and Feta (see page 306)

Lunch: Hearts of Palm and Tomato Salad (see page 276)

Dinner: Pork and Orzo Mediterranean Style

Servings: 6

Ingredients

- 1 ½ lbs. pork tenderloin
- 1 tsp. pepper
- 2 tbsp. olive oil
- 3 qt. water
- 1 ¼ cup orzo
- ¼ tsp. salt
- 6 oz. baby spinach, fresh
- 1 cup grape tomatoes, halved
- ¾ cup feta, crumbled

Directions

1. Massage pepper into pork. Cut into 1" cubes. Heat oil over medium heat in a large skillet. Add pork and cook until done.
2. In a Dutch oven, bring water to boil. Add in orzo and salt. Cook for 8 minutes, then add in spinach. Cook until orzo is al dente and spinach has wilted down. Drain.
3. Add tomatoes to skillet with pork and heat all the way through. Mix with orzo and add cheese.

Nutritional Facts
Calories: 372 | Carbs: 34g | Fat: 11g | Protein: 31g

DAY 25

Breakfast: Egg Muffins w/ Vegetable and Feta

Servings: 6

Ingredients

- 2 cups baby spinach, chopped
- ½ cup onion, chopped fine
- 1 cup tomatoes, chopped
- ½ cup kalamata olives, chopped
- 1 tbsp. oregano, fresh, chopped
- 2 tsp. sunflower oil
- 8 eggs
- 1 cup quinoa, cooked
- 1 cup feta, crumbled
- ¼ tsp. salt

Directions

1. Preheat oven to 350°F. Oil the muffin tins.
2. Heat skillet to medium heat and add in oil and onions. Cook until soft. Then, add in the tomatoes and cook for a minute. Now, add spinach and cook until wilted down. Remove from heat and add olives and oregano. Let sit.
3. Add eggs into a bowl and whisk until well combined. Then, add in cooked quinoa, feta, and vegetables. Mix and add salt.
4. Divide mixture evenly into muffin tin and bake for 30 minutes. Let cool and then serve.

Nutritional Facts
Calories: 114 | Carbs: 6g | Fat: 7g | Protein: 7g

Lunch: Lentil Patties w/ Mint Yogurt Sauce (see page 307)

Dinner: Olive, Caper, and Lemon Chicken (see page 313)

DAY 26

Breakfast: Frittata w/ Asparagus, Mushroom, & Goat Cheese (see page 230)

Lunch: Turmeric Cauliflower Soup

Servings: 6

Ingredients

- ¼ cup pumpkin seeds, raw
- 1 tsp. cumin, ground
- 2 tbsp. thyme, fresh, chopped
- 6 garlic cloves, chopped
- 2 cups onion, sliced
- 2 tbsp. olive oil
- 1 tbsp. turmeric
- 1 tbsp. flour, all-purpose
- 2 ½ cups chicken stock, unsalted
- ½ tsp. kosher salt
- 1 sm. head cauliflower, cut into florets
- 2 tsp. rice vinegar
- 3 tsp. brown sugar, light
- ½ tsp. pepper
- ¼ cup sour cream, light
- 2 tbsp. chives, fresh, chopped

Directions

1. Mix pumpkin seeds, cumin, and 1 ½ tsp. of oil in a bowl. Then, heat a skillet over medium heat and add mixture. Toast the mixture until lightly browned. Remove the mixture and set it to the side.

2. In a saucepan, heat 1½ tbsp. of oil over medium-high heat. Then, add onion, thyme, and garlic and cook until soft and fragrant. Then add turmeric and cook for another minute. Remove from heat.

3. Whisk in a bowl ½ cup of stock and the flour until combined. Add salt, cauliflower, and rest of stock to the saucepan. Heat over high heat and bring to boil. Lower the heat and simmer for 15 minutes.

4. Add this mixture into a food processor in batches and blend until smooth. Make sure to remove the center of the lid to release steam. When done, return to saucepan and stir in vinegar, sugar, and pepper. Cook for two minutes and then serve with pumpkin seeds, chives, and sour cream.

> *Nutritional Facts*
> *Calories: 149 | Carbs: 14g | Fat: 8g | Protein: 6g*

Dinner: Parmesan Pesto Tilapia (see page 263)

DAY 27

Breakfast: Poached Eggs with Greens & White Beans (see page 232)

Lunch: Sun-Dried Tomato & Feta Couscous Salad (see page 276)

Dinner: Spicy Mussels

Servings: 4

Ingredients

- 1 tbsp. olive oil, extra-virgin
- 1 tbsp. butter, unsalted
- 2 tbsp. shallot, chopped fine
- 1 oz. prosciutto, diced
- 2 tsp. garlic, chopped
- ½ tsp. red pepper flakes
- 1 cup tomatoes, chopped
- ½ cup white wine, dry
- 1 tsp. sugar
- ⅜ tsp. kosher salt
- 2 lbs. mussels, scrubbed and debearded
- 2 tbsp. parsley, fresh, chopped
- 2 lemons, wedged
- Whole baguette, sliced and toasted

Directions

1. Heat olive oil and butter over medium-high heat in a Dutch oven. Then add shallot and prosciutto. Cook until shallots are soft and prosciutto is crisp. Add garlic and pepper flakes and cook until garlic is fragrant. Add tomatoes, wine, sugar, and salt and simmer
2. Add mussels into the sauce. Cover and cook for appoximately 5 minutes until the mussels open. Serve in bowls with lemon wedges and crusty bread.

Nutritional Facts
Calories: 376 | Carbs: 26g | Fat: 10g | Protein: 38g

DAY 28

Breakfast: Mediterranean Eggs

Servings: 6

Ingredients

- 1 ½ lrg. onions, sliced
- 1 tbsp. butter
- 1 tbsp. olive oil, extra-virgin
- 1 garlic clove, minced
- ⅓ cup sun-dried tomatoes, drained, sliced
- 6-8 lrg. eggs
- 3 oz. feta, crumbled
- Salt and pepper for taste
- ⅓ cup parsley, fresh, chopped fine

Directions

1. Heat butter and oil in a cast-iron skillet over medium heat. Add in onions and cook until soft. Reduce heat and let onions cook for another 5-10 minutes until a soft brown color. Then, add garlic and sun-dried tomatoes and let cook until fragrant.
2. Spread the mix out until it is an even single layer on the bottom of the skillet. Crack eggs in skillet. Sprinkle the feta, salt, and pepper over the top. Cover skillet and cook for 10-15 minutes without removing the lid.
3. Remove pan from heat and sprinkle parsley over top, then serve.

Nutritional Facts
Calories: 183 | Carbs: 11g | Fat: 11g | Protein: 9g

Lunch: Tuna Melt w/ Olive Salsa (see page 301)

Dinner: Caprese Chicken (see page 292)

DAY 29

Breakfast: Avocado Toast Caprese Style (see page 229)

Lunch: Tomato Garlic Lentil Bowl

Servings: 6

Ingredients

- 1 tbsp olive oil
- 2 med. onions, chopped
- 4 garlic cloves, minced
- 2 cups dried lentils, brown, rinsed
- 1 tsp. salt
- ½ tsp. ginger, ground
- ½ tsp. paprika
- ¼ tsp. pepper
- 3 cups of water
- ¼ cup fresh lemon juice
- 3 tbsp. tomato paste
- ¾ cup Greek yogurt, fat-free, plain
- ⅓ cup cilantro, fresh, chopped

Directions

1. In a saucepan, heat oil over medium-high heat. Add onions and cook until soft. Then, add garlic and cook until it is fragrant. Stir in the lentils, seasoning, and water. Bring to a boil, then lower the heat and simmer covered for about 30 minutes.
2. Mix in the lemon juice and tomato paste and heat through. Serve with yogurt and cilantro.

Nutritional Facts
Calories: 294 | Carbs: 49g | Fat: 3g | Protein: 21g

Dinner: Honey Mustard Salmon (see page 264)

DAY 30

Breakfast: Start Your Morning Right Grain Salad (see page 234)

Lunch: Turmeric Cauliflower Soup (see page 314)

Dinner: Bruschetta Steak

Servings: 4

Ingredients

- 3 med. tomatoes, chopped
- 3 tbsp. basil, fresh, minced
- 3 tbsp. parsley, fresh, chopped
- 2 tbsp. olive oil
- 1 tsp. oregano, fresh, minced
- 1 garlic clove, minced
- ¾ tsp. salt
- 1 steak, flat-iron
- ¼ tsp. pepper
- ⅓ cup parmesan, grated

Directions

1. Combine tomatoes, basil, parsley, olive oil, oregano, and garlic. Add in ¼ tsp. salt and mix well. Then set to the side.
2. Season beef with pepper and salt after cutting in four pieces. Heat a grill pan over medium heat. Then, grill the steak to preferred doneness. Let rest and then top with tomato mixture. Sprinkle parmesan over the top and serve.

Nutritional Facts
Calories: 280 | Carbs: 4g | Fat: 19g | Protein: 23g

Disclaimer

The opinions and ideas of the author contained in this publication are designed to educate the reader in an informative and helpful manner. While we accept that the instructions will not suit every reader, it is only to be expected that the recipes might not gel with everyone. Use the book responsibly and at your own risk. This work with all its contents, does not guarantee correctness, completion, quality or correctness of the provided information. Always check with your medical practitioner should you be unsure whether to follow a low carb eating plan. Misinformation or misprints cannot be completely eliminated. Human error is real!

Design: Natalia Design

Printed in Great Britain
by Amazon